WE LIVED FOR THE BODY

WE LIVED

FOR THE BODY

Natural Medicine and Public
Health in Imperial Germany

AVI SHARMA

NIU Press
DeKalb, IL

© 2014 by Northern Illinois University Press
Published by Northern Illinois University Press, DeKalb, Illinois 60115

All Rights Reserved
Design by Yuni Dorr

Library of Congress Cataloging-in-Publication Data
Sharma, Avinash, author.
We lived for the body : natural medicine and public health in imperial Germany /
Avi Sharma.
pages cm
Includes bibliographical references and index.
ISBN 978-0-87580-704-1 (pbk.) — ISBN 978-1-60909-154-5 (e-book)
1. Naturopathy—Germany—History. 2. Public health—Germany—History. I. Title.
RZ440.S468 2014 615.5'350943—dc23
2014002289

CONTENTS

ACKNOWLEDGMENTS

I always expected the acknowledgments would be the easiest part of the book to write, but there are so many people who deserve my thanks for their help over the years. Michael Geyer, Leora Auslander, and Jan Goldstein all shaped the project in different ways and helped me to think through some difficult problems. Dan Koehler, Ari Joskowicz, Josh Arthurs, Joachim Haeberlen, Sean Forner, Ronen Steinberg, and Matt Calhoun were also there when this project began, and I am happy to say that I still get to see them here in Chicago, in Berlin, or elsewhere. We have had some pretty lively talks over the years, and I look forward to more conversations about German history and other important things.

While teaching at the University of Chicago, I had the chance to work with some outstanding people. John MacAloon and Chad Cyrenne directed the MAPSS program with both style and substance, and I was always so impressed by the way that they admired the young people they taught. I also had the chance to teach some amazing graduate students, now spread across the country. I expect many of them to make important contributions in their respective fields, but let me just mention a few who made a particular impact on my own thinking. David Chrisinger, Nina Arutyunyan, David Spreen, Claas Kirchhelle, Michaela Appeltova, Ciruce Movahedi-Lankarani, Ammar Ali Jan, and Clara Picker really captured my imagination at various points in our time together, and I look forward to reading their work as it comes out in the world.

I spent a fair bit of time doing research in Germany, and that was largely possible because of funding from the Fulbright Commission. Reiner Rohr was always an advocate for the Fellows, and he and his staff have done so much to support academic exchanges. I was a happy beneficiary of this excellent program.

The work would not have possible without the staff at libraries and archives in Germany and the United States. I am astonished at how much history is produced by the people working behind the scenes, and the generosity of people at the *Geheimes Staatsarchiv* and the *Staatsbibliothek* in Berlin, the *Hauptstaatsarchiv* in Dresden, and the Regenstein library in Chicago helped me to uncover materials that I am not sure I would have discovered on my own. Conferences organized by the Robert Bosch Institute for the History of Medicine, the Institute for Ethnology, and Institute for European History and Politics (both at Humboldt University), and the Center for Metropolitan Studies at the Technical University in Berlin all had a similar impact, introducing me to people and ideas that were new and exciting. In this regard, I want to thank Martin Dinges, Robert Jütte, Carsten Timmermann, Bo Sax, Harish Naraindas, Cornelia Regin, Volker Hess, Rainer Herrn, Beate Binder, Eric Engstrom. And then, of course, my special friends and mentors Dorothee Brantz and Thomas Mergel.

To Susan Bean, Amy Farranto, Judith Robey, Nancy Gerth, and Eric Miller, thank you for all the hard work you did putting this book together.

An earlier version of Chapter 2 was published in *Social History* 37 (2012): 36–54. An abbreviated version of Chapter 4 was published as "Medicine from the Margins? *Naturheilkunde* from Medical Heterodoxy to the University of Berlin, 1889–1921" in *Social History of Medicine* 24 (2011): 334–51. I also want to thank Robert Jütte and Martin Dinges for allowing me to use materials from "Rethinking Asymmetries in the Marketplace: Medical Pluralism in Germany, 1869–1910," in Martin Dinges, ed., *Medical Pluralism in Comparative Perspective: India and Germany, 1800–2000* (Stuttgart: Robert Bosch, 2014). My previous work is used here with permission.

Now for the many friends who have been so wonderful to me over the years. Kevin Royko, Aric Russom, Adam Buchwald, Ben Taylor, Kate Suisman, Genevieve Maull, Allan Lesage, Simen Strand, Lea Schleiffenbaum, Liza Weinstein, Allan Lesage, Matt Dorn, Ralf Bettermann, Imke Wagener, Ben Rubloff, Jenni Lee, Jana Obermuller, Julien Rouvroy, Antje Schnoor, Adam Levay, Dana Keiser, Karolina Gnatowski, Dan Gunn, Ben Helphand, Dawn Herrera, and many others have been so important to my experience, and I look forward to our continued conversation.

Most importantly, there is my family to thank. Gerda Neu-Sokol and Stephen Sokol are excellent second parents (I like this better than "in-laws"), and I love the conversations and arguments we have. Our relationship also has given me the chance to get to know the whole Neu-Simon clan, which has been a pleasure. My sister, Shalini, my mother Yasha, Berton, Arun, Navtej, Aleesha, Ayesha, Shail, Shashi, Shagun, Harneesh, Sohinee, Avinash, and Shaumya are all so valued by me. My father Yadu died just as this project was getting started, and my aunt Vasundhara (Basso) died as the book was just coming to an end. They are really missed by so many of us.

Finally, to my fascinating and lovely wife, Hannah. This would not have been nearly as interesting to me without you and the startling and surprising and funny conversations that we have. So thank you for that. Love you so much.

WE LIVED FOR THE BODY

INTRODUCTION
Progress Reconsidered: Natural Healing
and Germany's Long Nineteenth Century

Nature was central to the Wilhelmine experience. It organized medical cosmologies and reform initiatives; it informed consumer practices and lifestyle choices. Nature's appeal transcended class, confession, and political party. Kaiser Wilhelm II was an advocate for the "natural lifestyle," as was Karl Liebknecht, who announced the overthrow of Wilhelm's regime from the *Rote Rathaus* in 1918. Thomas Mann and Gerhardt Hauptmann thought that the "back-to-nature" mantra was evidence of a more or less severe psychological disorder, but Max Weber, who struggled with his own mental-health issues, was more forgiving and spent some time in a back-to-nature commune in Ascona. Millions of Germans—workers and bourgeois, aristocrats and industrialists—recognized that nature had healing effects and was intimately tied to quality-of-life issues. In the 1880s and 1890s, this preoccupation with nature became an increasingly important part of German popular culture. In organizations like the German League for Natural Lifestyle and Therapy, as well as in bathing, gymnastics, vegetarian, and land-reform groups, Germans from across the social and political spectrum claimed that nature was the key to imagining better futures.

In this book I explore the history of natural healing and show how popular health and hygiene movements shaped German ideas about nature in the long nineteenth century, from roughly 1800 to 1918. As Germans visited natural healers and submitted themselves to "natural" therapies, as they read manuals enjoining them to "get back to nature" and bought "reform" products that made it possible to live the "natural lifestyle," they increasingly experienced nature acting upon their own bodies and their everyday lives. During this time Germans tried to eat and drink "natural" foods. They exercised, bathed, sunned themselves, and spent time in the countryside, in forests, and in parks. They avoided university doctors offering "poisonous" medicines and worried about pollution near factories, overcrowding in cities, and the physical and moral dangers of urban poverty. Beginning in the 1880s—and over a period of several decades—nature, health, and the body became central to the way Germans talked about real and imagined social and political problems. This change in perspective had a variety of consequences and shaped the way that many people thought about their health, but also how they believed urban space should be used, doctors should be trained, children should be educated, and workers should be treated by their employers. The practice of popular medicine brought nature into urban daily life.

Historians have written little about the German natural healing movement, although a history of natural healing and popular medicine has important lessons for today. Recent decades have, for example, revealed growing anxieties about the quality of health care, about its social and economic costs, and about access to it. Concern about environmental degradation and long-term sustainability has also grown, particularly throughout Europe and North America. While environmentalism has developed in different ways in different parts of the world, sustainability has become a talking point for elected officials and activists across the globe.

Like the members of popular health and hygiene movements in Wilhelmine Germany, citizens today—on the left and right of the political spectrum, and on both sides of the Atlantic—are questioning the authority of scientific, corporate, and governmental actors to define the boundaries of civil, scientific, and economic discourse in contemporary society. In debates about vaccination, the prescription of mind-altering drugs to hyperactive children, and the production of Genetically Modified Organisms (GMOs)—as well as concerns about the pharmaceutical industry, animal cloning, and genetically modified foods—citizens are asking with ever-increasing frequency who has the authority to tell them what to believe about important scientific questions. In effect, they are testing the relationship between civil socity, the scientific community, and centers of state power.[1]

Health and hygiene reformers also debated access to quality health care, opportunities for sustainable development, the limits of parliamentary political process, and the relationship between scientists and the state. Looking back to the practice of popular medicine in Germany offers clues as to why certain practices—from community-based health solutions and rational urban planning to extraparliamentary political participation and popular health and science education—have today been pushed to the margins.

For decades historians have given scant attention to these issues,[2] but scholars of the nineteenth century have once again turned their attention to Germany's health and hygiene reform movements.[3] As part of the broader effort to think through "Wilhelminism and its Legacies,"[4] historians have tried to put the practice of popular medicine back into its contexts. Part of this is simply a numbers game. When historians in the 1990s started examining the natural healing movement and looking at data on membership numbers, institutional facilities, attendance at lectures, consumer habits, hospital visits, and insurance policies, it became increasingly clear that the practice of popular medicine—in particular, the natural healing movement—was not a phenomenon of the medical margins or political fringe.[5] As early as 1832, voluntary associations had been formed to celebrate the practice of Naturheilkunde (naturopathy),[6] and after the North German Trade Federation Act of 1869 freed the practice of medicine from restrictions of licensing and accreditation, Naturheilkunde came to occupy an increasingly prominent place in the medical marketplace. This period also saw the proliferation of natural healing associations and led to the creation in 1889 of the German League for Health Care and Nonmedicinal Healing Associations (Deutscher Bund der Vereine für Gesundheitspflege und arzneilose Heilweise).[7]

It has always been difficult to pin down the influence of the natural healing movement. We know, for example, that the German League

had roughly 19,000 members in 142 associations when it was founded, that this number grew to more than 148,000 members in some
890 local groups by 1914, and that the League's publicity organ, *Nature's Doctor (Naturarzt)*, was printing more than 160,000 copies per
issue at the beginning of the First World War.[8] These numbers are
not, however, entirely representative. For one thing, only the head of a
given household had to join the German League in order for the entire
family to use the League's facilities, which included libraries, access
to therapeutic instruments, bathing and sport facilities, and in some
cases, free medical consultation.

The German League was also part of a network of issue-oriented
reform movements—what contemporaries called the *Lebensreform*
movement—that shared institutional resources and often overlapped
in their personnel.[9] Important figures in the German League, for example, also occupied roles in societies focused on land reform, abstinence,
gymnastics, vegetarianism, nudism, suffrage, and opposition to vivisec-
tion. Oftentimes, entire associations would join the German League as
corporate members, expanding its representation significantly. Historian Florentine Fritzen tells us that, even in the 1920s and 1930s, when
membership in the German League was down by over 50 percent, the
constellation of Life-reform movements still counted more than 2 million Germans in its ranks,[10] and John Williams argues that, in part because of the controversies they generated, "naturist" movements had an
influence far out of proportion to their actual membership rolls. The
patronage of "prominent politicians and intellectuals, including Kaiser Wilhelm II, Friedrich Ebert, Karl Liebknecht, Getrud Baümer,
and many others," certainly contributed to the prominence of the
German League.[11] Nor was it just political activists who helped to
raise *Naturheilkunde's* profile: writers, painters, scientists, and social
reformers also played their part.[12]

No one can deny that race-nation extremists, back-to-the-land ro-
mantics, neopagan mystical types, and anti-Semites were *also* a part
of this culture of critical reform, and in a recent monograph, Chad
Ross argues that German nudism was closely tied to the rhetoric of
blood and soil, race and nation that became central to the National
Socialist campaign for power. Historians have shown, however, that

it would be wrong to assume that critical or oppositional groups existed only, or even primarily, at one or the other political or cultural extreme.[13] Martin Dinges, Florentine Fritzen, Robert Jütte, Cornelia Regin, John Williams, and Carsten Timmermann have all shown, for example, that in its criticisms of public health, housing, and hygiene, the natural healing movement developed a comprehensive reform agenda that included issues like a living wage, high-quality affordable housing, public-private partnerships for green belts and nature parks, tighter regulation of industrial waste, and federally mandated vacations for working men and women.[14] These critics have corrected the misconception that popular health and hygiene reform movements were confined to the historical margins, and they have shown just how influential this reform impulse was, particularly in the period between 1890 and 1918.

Nevertheless, whether or not this last generation of historians has succeeded in overturning the widespread perception that the natural healing movement *really was* backward-looking and conservative, or that it was somehow irrational and romantic (and therefore politically suspect)—is an entirely separate question. For their part, German historians have, by and large, rejected the facile logic that links a critique of an urban industrial modernity with romantic antimodernism, but they have not yet fully come to terms with the role these movements played in shaping the Wilhelmine experience. As we will see in subsequent chapters, health and hygiene reformers' ideas about a free medical marketplace, about the use of urban space, and about vaccination had the power to influence electoral outcomes, reverse ministry decisions, affect land-use policy, make millionaires, and shape the way individuals organized their everyday lives. Why, then, does the history of these ideas still remain on the margins of the discipline and the popular imagination? John Williams, Michael Hau, and others have researched natural healing, and their excellent work will be familiar to specialists. For a nonspecialist readership, though, natural healing—and the Life-reform movement more generally—remains an unfamiliar subject from the fringes of the German story.[15] This is not particularly surprising: after all, not a single English-language history of either natural healing or Life-reform has been published since World War I.

Part of the problem is a widespread misunderstanding of what natural healers and the millions who used their facilities, read their books, and bought their products were actually trying to accomplish. Unlike the allopathic medicine of the Wilhelmine period, *Naturheilkunde* was a holistic system that focused more on prevention than cures, more on everyday practices than on extraordinary illnesses. Natural healers and Life-reformers were not only interested in disease and treatment. Theirs was a holistic medical cosmology, a critique of Wilhelmine urban industrial modernity, and a way of introducing nature into the urban experience. Natural healing was always about more than just medicine. Members of the German League were articulating alternative ways of thinking about public health, urban spaces, and individual choice.

Unless we try to understand the German natural healing movement by looking at how it viewed itself, we confine ourselves to quirky narratives based upon misconceptions about healers practicing their art in an unenlightened age.[16] In this kind of account, the movement's holistic critique of urban industrial modernity disappears entirely. However, understanding *Naturheilkunde's* history on its own terms is no easy task. It is only possible if we first think seriously about how we compare different healing traditions and what we mean when we think and talk about progress. Such an undertaking will require a brief detour through (the politics of) German historiography.

WHAT IS AT STAKE IN RETHINKING "PROGRESS"

German historiography has been a peculiar affair for decades, and that is the case because so much of it was written in order to explain how things went so very wrong. In the period between roughly 1950 and 1980, historians wanted to understand how Germany could have been so "modern" in its industry, academic institutions, and economic infrastructure yet at the same time have been so politically and culturally retrograde. This generation of historians was writing during the heyday of early modernization theorists like Walt Rostow and Samuel Huntington, who argued that there were objective metrics for determining successful and failed development.

More democracy, more open markets, more social mobility, more science, more technology, more urbanization—all were taken as indicators of an increasing degree of modernization. Germany's story was, in this sense, a particular iteration of a global discourse. The German road to National Socialism was a cautionary tale about the consequences of the failure to fully modernize.[17] The German case was also politically expedient during the Cold War: in a divided Europe, it was one more example of the terrible things that could happen when the people rejected democracy, or when they turned to the state instead of toward markets. Now this is a thumbnail sketch, and a crude one at that,[18] but the key point is that German history was written using the discourse of progress and pathology. Analyzing events in German history using these normative concepts has important consequences.

I am not suggesting anything new here. Historians, sociologists, anthropologists, and others have written extensively about the problems—from ethnocentrism to historical determinism—that plague modernization theory and the metaphors of progress and pathology that are at its ethical core. Geoff Eley and David Blackbourn played a major role in dismantling the so-called *Sonderweg* hypothesis, which cited Germany's "special path" to modernity as the cause of its pathologies. Their work helped to usher in generations of new scholarship that focused more on historical plurality than on the essentially normative perspective that underpinned modernization narratives.[19] For decades now, historians have been explicit in rejecting "modernization" theory in favor of a more pluralistic understanding of our own recent histories.[20]

If historians have largely rejected the metaphor of progress in thinking about political or cultural history, though, *this is not necessarily true when it comes to histories of medicine, science, and technology*. In his otherwise excellent book *The Cult of Health and Beauty*, Michael Hau tells us, for example, that medical cosmologies like *Naturheilkunde* were really just an attempt to simplify medicine so that the simple people could understand it. Despite the fact that natural healers explicitly *celebrated* the simplicity of their holistic therapies, even some of the best historians continue to suggest that natural healers may have turned to their craft because they could not keep up with the medical "state of the art."[21] *Naturheilkunde* was, in this view, a survivor of older medical cosmologies that had since been superseded by new medical technologies. To put it another way, natural healing and Life-reform remained stuck in the past, while conventional medicine marched into the modern era. This interpretation has important political effects that ultimately shape our everyday lives. I will elaborate upon this point in the forthcoming chapters.

It turns out that historians are perfectly willing to do away with the metaphor of progress when writing social, cultural, or political histories (after all, who wants to be the one claiming that Europeans "have progressed more than" or "are more modern than" Africans, Asians, Americans, or Australians?) even as many of us continue to operate as though "Medicine" and "Science" *are* progressive, and will, over time, continue to advance toward an undisclosed goal. How does one explain this inconsistency? Historian of science Peter Dear suggests that our faith in Science can only be explained if we understand that science is really made up of two distinct components: it is a way of seeing the physical world, and it is also a way of controlling the physical world. Thus, when the "scientific worldview" falls short of its promise to explain the physical world or to improve the human experience, we remind ourselves of technological triumphs—space travel, microprocessors, antiviral cocktails, genetic sequencing, prosthetics, nuclear technology, and bunker-busting bombs—that seem to prove that *science works*. When science as technology (or, as Dear puts it, "power over matter") fails us, we are referred to the promise of science in its abstract form. When, for example, atomic bombs level Hiroshima and Nagasaki or bacteria do not respond to standard treatment protocols, we remember that the "scientific worldview" is also charting the mysteries of the universe and explaining why the planet is warming. The point is that, when it comes to "science," there are myriad reasons to believe that "Progress" as a category might in fact be real.[22] If modernization theory is on its way out, as historians Michael Geyer and Konrad Jarausch suggest, its deep metaphor—progress—appears to be alive and well when it comes to the fields of Science, Technology, and Medicine. Perhaps we have not moved beyond modernization as much as we claim to have done.

To truly move beyond the structural core of the modernization narrative, it is essential that we begin to take seriously insights generated by historians, sociologists, and philosophers of science. In dozens of important works over the last three decades, scholars like Bruno Latour, Steve Shapin, Thomas Gieryn, Peter Dear, Corinna Treitel, Carsten Timmerman, Robert Johnston, and James Whorton have shown how *even science* is produced through particular laboratory processes, political conjunctures, funding structures, publicity campaigns, and personal relationships.[23] In other words, science is no different from other fields of human endeavor, where "progress" can only be defined as the movement toward a *particular* goal.

Rethinking progress is important because it is a first step in seriously engaging with the practice of popular medicine on its own terms, rather than as a vestige of an earlier age. In the process, new kinds of histories begin to emerge: these are histories where lay persons participated differently in conversations about public health and urban planning than they do now, and where the links between inequality and morbidity were recognized not just by epidemiologists, but also by those populations most directly affected by those issues. By taking seriously the practice of popular medicine, we can start to think about history as open-ended, and about modernity as a contested field.

The arguments critiquing the notion of progress in the history and philosophy of science are fairly abstract, so I will offer a concrete example. When asked about popular protest against compulsory smallpox vaccination in the *fin de siècle*, I always run up against the fact that smallpox, as a naturally occurring phenomenon, was eradicated by the World Health Organization's postwar global vaccination campaign. Does that not mean, I am often asked, that the vaccinators were right, and the anti-vaccine agitators were wrong?[24] Is the eradication of smallpox not evidence that conventional medicine is superior to natural healing, and that science is, indeed, progressive?

That is certainly one way to look at it. It seems to me equally important, though, that we start to ask other questions. What, for example, would the public health system look like if it were organized around prevention, public works, and efficient administrative and policing institutions to control the outbreak of infectious diseases?[25] The triumph of the WHO campaign against smallpox taught us, among other things, that you can eradicate disease without doing very much about the social contexts in which it spreads.[26] Over a period of decades, the WHO campaign shaped the way that relief and medical resources were deployed, particularly in colonial and postcolonial contexts, where governmental and nongovernmental efforts came increasingly to focus on pharmaceutical intervention, oftentimes at the expense of infrastructure, education, and community care facilities. Perhaps nineteenth-century critics of compulsory vaccination were right to argue that the search for silver bullets was a sure-fire way to make policymakers and the public complacent in addressing the root causes of disease.[27]

Those skeptical of my line of reasoning might be surprised to hear what the National Institutes of Health have to say about the whole thing. Their 2001 report suggests that "compared to mass vaccination, surveillance and containment are thought to have provided more effective means of controlling the spread of smallpox disease."[28] There is no doubt that the WHO campaign succeeded in eradicating smallpox as a naturally occurring disease. But the question remains: What opportunities were lost, and what were the costs?[29] These are some of the questions raised by Life-reformers during the Wilhelmine era. When they tried to overturn an 1874 compulsory vaccination law, they were not just proposing using natural therapies to combat smallpox: they were imagining a future where public health and individual practices were all organized differently. Recognizing the alternative futures imagined by Wilhelmine reformers is only really possible, though, if we start to put into practice those things that we generally agree about in theory: that science, too, is social, and that progress is not actually an analytical category. By taking seriously the work of historians, sociologists, and philosophers of science, we can finally put to rest the deep metaphor of the modernization theory that so many of us explicitly disavow. This book is an attempt to recover the holistic approach to health and healing that made Naturheilkunde distinctive. In the process, I hope to recover some of those futures imagined by Life-reformers in the nineteenth and early twentieth centuries.

Chapter 1 is called "Creating Nature's Republic: From Natural Therapies to Self-Help in Germany, 1800–1870." It looks at how the theory and practice of Naturheilkunde changed in the first several decades of the nineteenth century. Starting with charismatic healers like Vincenz Prießnitz in the beginning of the nineteenth century, and ending with the creation of new preventive and therapeutic technologies just before German unification, I show how "nature" organized *Naturheilkunde* across a period of many decades. If *nature* was central to how lay healers mediated social practice, it was also a category constantly in flux. As medical theory changed, as therapeutic practices evolved, and as the audience for natural therapies expanded, the category "nature" was itself transformed. By the 1870s, nature was becoming a model not just for "the cure" but also for organizing everyday lives. This chapter shows the role of changing medical theories and practices in shaping the category "nature."

In the second chapter, "Wilhelmine Nature: Natural Lifestyle and Practical Politics in the German Life-Reform Movement, 1890–1914," I show how the medico-therapeutic model associated with *Naturheilkunde* became the foundation for a broad-based social movement. Focusing on the formation of new consumer publics, and the rapid expansion of association culture, I show how a complex of nature concepts began to circulate far from the contexts of their creation. In bathing facilities and association halls, retail outlets and urban-reform initiatives, "nature" became one of the defining concepts of the Wilhelmine era.

In the third chapter, "Contesting the Medical Marketplace: Politics, Publicity, and Scientific Progress, 1869–1910," I show how alternative medicine in general, and natural healing in particular, fits into the German medical landscape. After 1869, when the North German Trade Federation Act freed the practice of medicine from requirements of education and accreditation, nonlicensed natural healers entered the medical marketplace in ever greater numbers. Licensed doctors and the professional organizations that represented doctors' interests tried to define their competitors as charlatans, swindlers, and quacks, and they supported numerous legislative efforts to force their nonlicensed colleagues from the marketplace. Natural healers and the associations formed to protect their professional interests were, predictably enough, vocal in their defense of the free medical marketplace. But my main focus is on the newspaper editors and police officials, the lawyers, parliamentarians, and even doctors who came out in defense of the free medical marketplace. The efforts of all of these different agents on behalf of natural healers offer us insights not only into the way that contemporaries thought about civil liberties and individual rights, but also the way that they imagined scientific progress and the role of experts in society.

My fourth chapter is called "Science from the Margins? *Naturheilkunde* from Outsider Medicine to the University of Berlin, 1889–1920." It examines issues of boundary definition between *Naturheilkunde* and academic medicine by showing how natural therapies were absorbed into the medical mainstream at the same time that medical men tried to exclude lay practitioners from the professional practice of medicine. This kind of boundary work shifted course repeatedly between 1880 and roughly 1920. I argue that, in the end, *Naturheilkunde* was itself transformed by the institutionalization of its practices. This institutionalization goes some way in explaining why more than 70 percent of the Germans canvassed in 1992 claimed to have used natural therapies (*Naturheilverfahren*) at some point in their careers and why such a significant percentage of German doctors specialize or have sub-specialties in natural healing.[30]

In my final chapter, "Anti-Vaccine Agitation, Parliamentary Politics, and the State in Germany, 1874–1914," I explore popular resistance to compulsory vaccination from its introduction in 1874 to the eve of the First World War. In chapters 2 through 4 the core themes were nature, the consumer public and popular culture, civic freedoms, and science and its definition. In this chapter, I bring all of those themes together in an attempt to understand the variety of reasons people had for resisting smallpox vaccination and the strategies they deployed in their efforts. Smallpox was, of course, eradicated in 1979/1980, and so it may seem natural to assume that vaccine advocates were "right" and vaccine resisters were "wrong." In this chapter, I argue that this is the wrong way to frame the problem. Vaccine advocates and vaccine critics were all making a series of positive claims—not just about how smallpox works, about technologies to control it, and about how to organize public health. They were also making assertions about the unintended consequences of vaccine-induced immunity, about the kinds of responsibilities individuals should have for ensuring their own health and well-being, and about what society should look like. It is this positive project that deserves our attention.

We Lived for the Body is about how natural healing developed, survived, and thrived in Germany between roughly 1800 and 1918. The first part of the book charts the evolution of natural healing, showing how it became a holistic medical cosmology concerned not just with the cure but also with the urban everyday, not just with individuals but also with the body social. In chapters 1 and 2, I show how the theory and practice of *Naturheilkunde* changed over a period of about 120 years, and I also explore how the practice of popular medicine helped to change what it was that Germans meant when they talked about "nature."

The second part of the book explores how *Naturheilkunde* became implicated in different aspects of German public life in the period between roughly 1874 and 1920. Part 2 certainly addresses the relationship between nonlicensed healers and the medical establishment, but it is about far more than just a contest between competing medical practices or professional interest groups. In the chapters about the "free medical marketplace," the institutionalization of natural therapies in the German academy, and resistance to compulsory vaccination in the period after 1874, I show how the holistic ideas that were so central to *Naturheilkunde* were grafted onto a range of other debates and ultimately shaped German ideas about nature, health, and the body.

CHAPTER ONE

CREATING NATURE'S REPUBLIC

From Natural Therapies to Self-Help

in Germany, 1800–1870

In the nineteenth century, natural healers claimed that "nature" (and not doctors) was responsible for health and healing. The healers argued that water cures and dietary practices could restore the sick person to health, while the medications prescribed by allopathic doctors addressed symptoms rather than the patient. The emphasis on the healing power of nature was a consistent feature of natural healing throughout the nineteenth century, and this sometimes creates the impression that natural healing did not change very much during that period. In the late nineteenth and early twentieth centuries, medical associations tried to foster this view, claiming that natural healers recycled archaic therapies while academic medicine was making progress through laboratory research.[1] If one focuses on therapeutic practices, as medical men did, it does sometimes seem that natural healers were more conservative in their response to new treatments than their allopathic colleagues were. By shifting the focus from particular therapies to a more comprehensive view of natural healing, though, we get a different perspective.

This chapter explores how natural healing evolved over the course of the nineteenth century to become a holistic medical cosmology more concerned with prevention than with cures, more focused on health than sickness, and more interested in social practices than symptoms. Exploring how natural healing changed over the nineteenth century helps to explain why natural healers were so concerned with the everyday behaviors of their patients, and why their prescriptions were so different from those of their allopathic colleagues. "Nature" is central to this story because from the beginning of the nineteenth century to the end, natural healers claimed that only "nature" could heal. To understand the evolution of natural healing over the course of the century, then, we have to look at what natural healers meant when they talked about nature.

Telling this story is no easy task, in part because "nature" itself is so difficult to define. In the very useful collection *Germany's Nature*, for example, "nature" is used to signify a place or a divine presence. It is used as a noun (as in "technology is not alien to nature") and as an adjective (as in "natural man" or "natural landscape").[2] Other sources look at the concept of nature as a force. Historian John Williams, for example, claims that nature was defined "as an antidote to urban industrial modernity,"[3] while Uwe Heyll tells us that "[the] idea of a healthful nature was not new," but had been around since antiquity.[4] Historians have pointed to different genealogies of the nature concept. In the late eighteenth and early nineteenth centuries, for example, German speakers consistently referred to nature as an abstract ideal and a space untainted by human hands. German romanticism is also cited for its role in evangelizing nature.[5] In the history of medicine, it is common to cite a different trajectory, from Hippocrates to Galen, and then, centuries later, to Christoph Wilhelm Hufeland.[6] Nature meant different things in different contexts. In tracing the evolution of natural healing across the nineteenth century, I show one important way that German ideas about nature were formed.[7]

This chapter shows how the practice of popular medicine helped to change the way that nature was understood by contemporaries. In the hands of natural healers, nature was not the transcendental, quasi-religious ideal offered by romantic poets, nor was it simply the opposite of urban space. Over the course of the nineteenth century, as natural healers tried to use nature to improve their patients' health, they began to talk about nature as an example to be followed and a tool that could transform individual lives. As natural healers began to focus more on preventive medicine than on "the cure" and more on the everyday habits of their patients than on their immediate symptoms, they helped to transform how nature was defined and understood. Theirs was not, of course, the only definition. Poets continued to refer to nature's transcendental beauty, nature was often used to refer to nonurban landscapes, and cultural critics still spoke of unspoiled nature as an antidote to degeneracy. As natural healers used nature as a model for everyday practices and as a tool to combat sickness, though, nature also came to mean something less abstract. In part through the practice of popular medicine, nature slowly became a way to organize one's daily life.

This trajectory might be just another interesting genealogy of a complex concept, but in this chapter and the next, I argue that it was something more than that. These chapters show that the practice of popular medicine helped to preserve ideas about nature that were losing traction in other areas of public life. For much of the eighteenth century, and into the nineteenth, nature figured prominently in a range of fields, from literature and philosophy to commerce and medicine. This began to change in the period after roughly 1830, particularly as romanticism and *Naturphilosophie* declined in their influence. But if nature was losing its defining significance in the first decades of the nineteenth century, how does one explain its renaissance in popular and consumer cultures in the period between 1890 and 1918, a period when it sometimes seemed that everyone—from the members of youth groups to bureaucrats in the ministry of the interior—was talking about nature?[8]

This chapter shows that natural healing helped to preserve a range of ways of thinking and talking about nature, precisely at a time when these ideas were losing their significance in many other fields of German life. Until well after German unification in 1871, these ideas remained confined to a relatively small population of those dedicated to the theory and practice of natural healing. But this changed dramatically during the Wilhelmine era, when natural healing exploded in popularity. By the end of the nineteenth century, natural healers and lifestyle entrepreneurs had introduced a domesticated version of nature into the everyday lives of millions of Germans, both inside and outside of the natural healing movement. In the hands of natural healers, nature was transformed into a model for everyday living, and not just an abstract ideal. If one wants to understand why nature figured so centrally in

Wilhelmine conversations on everything from health and hygiene to city planning and labor law, the transformation of popular medicine offers important clues.[9]

Tracking the trajectory of natural healing over a period of several decades can also help us to understand the popular reception of the hygiene sciences in German-speaking lands, because as natural healers increasingly focused on the importance of lifestyle and preventive health care, they also helped to popularize protohygienic discourses that stressed both individual responsibility *and* social reform. Historians have typically argued that hygiene discourse was pioneered in universities, medical associations, and state bureaucracies—and that this discourse was spread by bourgeois social reformers.[10] Instead of the top-down perspective offered by some historians, my account suggests how popular cultures can help us to understand the way that German public health evolved. For the reading public and in Germany's flourishing association culture, new ways of defining nature found their way into the popular lexicon. The idea that nature could be a model not just for healing, but also for everyday living is one reason that protohygienic discourse about lifestyle and prevention achieved such broad circulation. This development helps to explain the popular reception of health and hygiene discourse in German popular culture in the final decades of the nineteenth century.

This chapter focuses on an idea and the transformation of that idea through the theory and practice of natural healing. It is not intended as a comprehensive look at the medical-therapeutic landscape between 1800 and 1871, even though a study of that sort would no doubt be useful. The first part of the chapter explores the work of the natural healer Vincenz Prießnitz in the first decades of the nineteenth century, highlighting the way that he used nature as a model for his therapies. In the second part of the chapter, I examine how a narrow focus on water cures among natural healers was supplanted by a more holistic approach to health and healing that used nature as a model not just for therapy, but also for everyday living. Ultimately, I hope to show how the transformation of natural healing over a period of several decades changed what it was that nature meant to historical actors. As nature became a model not just for the cure, but also for day-to-day living, it also became part of a broader conversation about health, hygiene, and preventive practice.

WATER CURES: NATURE AS A MODEL FOR THERAPEUTIC PRACTICE

Most histories of natural healing in German-speaking lands start, rightly, with Vincenz Prießnitz (1799–1851). Considered by many to be the father of *Naturheilkunde*, Prießnitz grew up on a small landholding in Gräfenberg bei Freiwaldau in Austrian Silesia.[11] Reports about his upbringing vary. While we know that he was raised Catholic, there is little information about his childhood or his education. One historian, Christian Andree, claims that, despite intensive archival exploration, he was unable to authenticate a single document signed by the famous healer.[12] Some sources suggest that Prießnitz was likely to have been only semiliterate. He was the son of a small landholder in the early nineteenth century, so his school attendance would probably have been sporadic at best.[13] Decades after his death, the natural healing movement actually celebrated the fact that Prießnitz likely never passed beyond grammar school. As lay healers tried to defend their right to practice their therapies against those who wanted to exclude them from a medical marketplace, Prießnitz was used to justify the work of "other healers" who had nothing to offer except their native abilities and their experiences.[14] Citing Prießnitz as an example, they claimed that instinct and experience, not university training, provided the true measure of a healer. While some critics of natural healing contested that interpretation, even they were unable to deny that Prießnitz was a master of his craft.[15]

The stories describing Prießnitz's discovery of water therapies often used a quasi-religious language, and historians have picked up on this. In his very worthwhile study of natural healing, for example, Uwe Heyll has chapters entitled "The Paradise of Health" and "From Religion to Utopia," while Eva Barlösius claims that advocates of natural healing often described their advocacy as the end result of their "conversion" from mainstream therapies.[16] In one popular version, the young Prießnitz came upon a wounded stag bathing at a forest watering hole.[17] He remembered the stag years later, in 1816, when he himself was injured (he sustained multiple rib fractures while trying to quiet a team of horses). Unable to find a doctor to set the broken ribs, Prießnitz attempted to heal himself,[18] by first leaning against a chair and breathing deeply to reset the bones, and then binding his chest using a moist cloth, secured with a tight dry wrap. Prießnitz used the least invasive procedure available to get his body back to normal. Known in lay and medical circles as the "Prießnitz Compress," the wrap secured the bone and controlled swelling. According to all accounts, he recovered quickly.[19] In future accounts, his 1816 experience is cited as a turning point: it was the moment when he was converted to natural therapies.

For some, this story about an illiterate boy who saw nature as a model for healing showed that instinct and native ability were more important than medical degrees and state licenses. Eduard Schnitzlein, himself a medical doctor, claimed in an 1838 pamphlet on water therapies that Prießnitz was a doctor by instinct. "As it is given to the artist to develop within himself the fullness of harmony and tone . . . so it is with Prießnitz, who has been given a knowledge of sickness, who can confidently judge the life force of the individual, who can perceive in his deep and true gaze the organic processes of life itself."[20] Prießnitz may have had an intuitive understanding of his craft, but he also consciously used nature as a model for his therapies. These natural therapies found a ready audience. At the age of 19, Prießnitz was performing cures as far away as Bohemia and Mähren, and by 1822, he had to build several cottages on his property to accommodate the ever-growing number of cure seekers. Over the years, Prießnitz developed an elaborate system of water therapy comprised of 56 different procedures that included cold-water and steam baths, cold compresses, and sweat-inducing wraps.[21] What were Prießnitz cures like, and what did patients experience when arriving at Gräfenberg?[22]

One of the first things new guests experienced at Gräfenberg was a cold bath. Ranging from 17–20 degrees Réaumur (62.6–68 degrees Fahrenheit), the bath was the basis for a preliminary diagnosis. The patient's reactions to the chilly water determined whether he or she was ready to begin a full treatment, or whether preliminary work was required. Prießnitz was always present for this intake, and if the patient failed to show a vigorous blush, he or she would continue with daily cool water baths until sufficiently "toughened" for therapies that became more and more intense over the course of the patient's stay.

The full cure was made up of a seemingly unending schedule of bathing, showers, steam, and sitting. At four in the morning, guests were wakened, wrapped in woolen comforters intended to make them sweat, and returned to their beds. Those patients suffering from skin complaints—for example, eczema, syphilitic sores, or boils—were each wrapped first in a damp linen sheet and then in a woolen comforter (*Leintuch*). This was meant to stimulate the skin and to purify the body by initiating intensive sweating. Once patients had begun to sweat, bathing attendants opened the windows to let in fresh, cool air and compelled the guests to drink glass after glass of cold water.

After 30 to 60 minutes, patients entered bathtubs filled with cold water heated to a range of six to eight degrees Réaumur (45.5–50 degrees Fahrenheit), significantly colder than the water used at the intake examinations. Fresh spring water was regularly added, and dirty water was siphoned off. The length of the bath depended on the sensitivity of the patient, but it typically lasted between six and eight minutes. Having evaluated the patients' overall fitness through the initial phases of treatment, Prießnitz prescribed different combinations of partial and full baths, body wraps, and massages, all designed to stimulate and strengthen the body's regulatory systems. In addition to cleansing the body of harmful toxins, improving circulation and respiration, the combination of wraps and water therapies was thought to toughen and invigorate (*abhärten*) the whole body. Upon completing this alternating routine of sweating and cold bathing, patients were sent walking to raise the body temperature naturally.

At approximately nine in the morning, a full five hours after waking, guests ate a light breakfast consisting of cold milk and dark bread. The guests then made the 30-minute trek to outdoor showers (five of which were for men and three for women) located above the facilities at the so-called *Hirschbadkamm*, where Prießnitz first had his revelation while observing the stag. This walk after breakfast was supposed to have salutary effects, stimulating muscles and respiration, but in cases where the patients were unable to make the journey, there were ox-drawn wagons available to transport them. The showers reserved for men were vigorous, even violent, with water at a temperature of five degrees Réaumur

(43.25 degrees Fahrenheit) falling from a height of four meters. These showers (*Sturzbäder*), lasting anywhere between two and five minutes, were intended to shock the system and to toughen it up. While Andree does not report on the female showers, one would imagine that they were based upon a similar principle, though adjusted for the perceived sensitivities of women.

After the showers and a vigorous walk back to the facilities, the guests were served lunch. This main meal of the day typically included a variety of meat dishes, breads, and starches. Vegetables were rarely served. Prießnitz typically joined his guests during this lunch hour, encouraging them to eat heartily and to imbibe heroic amounts of fresh, cold, spring water. After lunch, the guests were directed either to more sweat-inducing wraps or to partial baths. Stimulating particular areas of the skin was thought to be one way to act on inner organs and regulatory systems. Stimulating the nerves in the skin on the arms and chest, for example, was thought to increase the flow of blood to the lungs and heart, while stimulating the feet through heat or cold was said to affect the mucous membranes in the nose. Thus, Prießnitz might have ordered sweat-inducing wraps for illnesses like asthma and diabetes, while prescribing cold baths to calm patients prone to sleeplessness or severe headaches.[23] In the afternoon, each guest would either return to the showers, or go walking again, this time wrapped in a "Neptune belt," which consisted of a moist sheet wrapped around the stomach and genitals and secured by a dry towel. At seven in the evening, dinner—which, like breakfast, consisted of dark bread and cold milk—was served. Guests were encouraged to retire shortly after nine o'clock.[24]

Through this cure and others like it, his reputation as a healer grew rapidly, spreading by word of mouth across the region. In 1829, the Gräfenberg sanatorium hosted 49 guests. Ten years later, the number of guests had grown to 1,780.[25] Although Prießnitz's annual income is contested, Jürgen Helfricht claims that the healer's fortune exceeded 200,000 Gulden. This can be usefully compared with the income of the city of Freiwaldau for the year 1845, which was roughly 13,000 Gulden.[26] By the beginning of the 1840s, tales about the miraculous Prießnitz cure were being cited as far away as England and America as evidence of the superiority of the water cure.[27] It is said that the famous "water doctor" once received a letter from America that was addressed to "Vincenz Prießnitz in Europe."[28] These details are certainly suggestive, but who were his guests, why did they come, and what was their experience like? A variety of sources—guides to the Gräfenberg cure, memoirs, and propaganda pieces—offer a partial answer to these questions.

In 1839, roughly 120 of the cure-seekers were medical doctors.[29] In 1845, the Archduke Franz Karl of Austria visited. At the same time, the Duchess of Anhalt-Köthen, the Archbishop from Breslau Melchior von Diepenbrock, the King of Saxony, Chopin, and the Head of the Order of Jesuits P. Bexx were all in residence.[30] At the time of his visit in 1841, the Englishman R. T. Claridge claimed that "there are under his treatment an archduchess, ten princes and princesses, *at least* one hundred counts and barons, military men of all grades, several medical men, professors, advocates and others."[31] On the surface, Gräfenberg could have been a spa like those in the famous towns of Central and Eastern France or southwest Germany, catering to the European nobility and celebrating hierarchies of rank and distinction.

Prießnitz tried to create a different atmosphere at his sanatorium, where health—not hierarchy—was on display. One visitor remarked that, even though the "highest and richest nobility in Europe visited Gräfenberg,"[32] every effort was made to insure that an egalitarian sensibility prevailed, with each new guest without exception taking the place farthest from Prießnitz ["*den untersten Platz*"] in the dining room.[33] The famous French historian Jules Michelet (1798–1874) went further, writing that "after the Bacchanalia of the Restoration, we saw Prießnitz impose the heaviest penance on Europe's grand aristocracy. They dined on farmers' bread, while the most sensitive ladies bathed under ice-cold water in the dead of winter. So great is mans' love for life, so great his fear of death, and his reverence for nature. As soon, that is, as he feels his strength leaving him."[34] At Gräfenberg, the desire for health trumped vanity.

It was not just in matters of rank that a peculiarly free atmosphere prevailed, as the testimony of one guest indicates: "It should be easy to see that in such circumstances, given the guests' great interest in the cure, the conversation often turned on topics that simply were not spoken of in cultivated circles. In Gräfenberg one might speak with a woman about sweating, bathing, eruptions and abscesses, and, though only in lowered tones, even about enemas (*Klystiere*)....At first, new guests were quite shocked by this freedom [of speech], but realized quickly that at Gräfenberg, we lived only for the body."[35] No doubt in questions of rank as in those of gender, distinctions were made and boundaries were drawn. It does, however, appear that guests submitted to a modified set of social norms at Gräfenberg and, in doing so, submitted to the will of the peasant healer Vincenz Prießnitz.

In some ways, Gräfenberg was part of a larger spa culture that was popular in Europe, England, and, to a lesser extent, the United States. Gräfenberg, like spas across Europe, was staffed by bathing attendants and medical doctors who were responsible for overseeing therapy; the schedule was rigidly organized; and bath, steam, and drinking waters were considered to be powerful healing tools. Taking the cure also frequently meant a major break from day-to-day life. While some patients, particularly those with limited financial resources, went for brief visits, it was common to stay for extended periods of time, in many cases, for longer than one month. The cure, whether at the baths of Gräfenberg, Aix, or Vichy, was an extraordinary event, and this seems to have been part of the reason for its effectiveness: guests focused, more or less effectively, on their health.

If Gräfenberg was in some respects similar to Europe's more famous spas, it was also very different. Its geographic isolation and rigorous regimen served to indicate the attitude that prevailed at Prießnitz's facilities: patients rose earlier and endured waters that were far colder than at comparable spas in Central and Western Europe. They were served coarse peasant food. Gambling and alcohol were forbidden, and instead of walking along boulevards through the town, they were directed to the forests and parks around Gräfenberg.[36] Another factor seems to have been peculiar to Gräfenberg. While the grand spas of Europe put wealth and power on display, Prießnitz tried to subordinate the status of his patients to the dictates of their treatment regimens.[37] It is impossible to say why so many thousands visited Gräfenberg. But as Michelet pointed out in 1861, they were all willing to entrust their bodies and their health to a barely literate peasant whose chief claim to competence was his particular ability to understand and to see the laws of nature at work. Perhaps his patients really did "live for the body."

Prießnitz and the various patients, guests, observers, acolytes, and critics who wrote about his life and work all shared a variety of assumptions about nature, health, and healing.[38] But that is not the same as saying that they shared the same conception of nature itself. In fact, they drew on a variety of sources for their conceptions of nature: philosophical ideas (like Rousseau's injunction to return to nature); medical traditions (whether Galenic or Hippocratic); and religious or quasi-religious ideas of nature.

These are all different trajectories for a particular view of nature, and they all, no doubt, warrant our attention. For present purposes, though, it is most important to note what these views had in common. From all of these perspectives, nature was a book that one would do well to read, and it was worth reading because it was as deeply rational as it was essentially good. Reading nature meant seeing with clear eyes, listening to one's instincts, being open to the examples offered by the natural world, and remembering that nature, not the doctor, has the power to heal. This perspective was popularized, in part, by Prießnitz's most famous student, Johannes Rausse. In Rausse's hands, though, the water therapies offered by Prießnitz were slowly transformed into a holistic system that was concerned with prevention and not just with "the cure." In the process, nature was reimagined as a model for daily living, rather than an ideal to be emulated at the spas of Europe. The individual slowly moved to the center of this model, replacing the figure of the great healer.

PREVENTION: FROM THE CURE TO EVERYDAY PRACTICES

In his 1796 *Art of Prolonging Life*, Christoph Wilhelm Hufeland, personal physician to Goethe and Professor of Medicine at the University of Berlin, told his readers that sickness and health existed along a continuum. From birth until death, all humans are more or less sick and expend their life force with each moment.[39] This was not a particularly controversial claim: according to Howard Kaye, the idea that sickness was different from health in degree rather than kind had, by the 1850s, "long since achieved the status of dogma, not only in physiology and medicine . . . but . . . in philosophy[,] psychology[,] and sociology . . . as well."[40] On the surface, this may seem like a point hardly worthy of notice, but it was the necessary, if not sufficient, condition for the emergence of the hygiene sciences. Prevention, and not the cure, was the key to this idea of health along a continuum. This perspective was popularized, in part, by Rausse.

Philo vom Walde calls Rausse the "first *scientific* founder of *Wasserheilkunde*,"[41] and it is not hard to see why he thought this might be the case.[42] Although few doubted Prießnitz's instinct for healing, he never articulated a systematic healing philosophy. Rausse, on the other hand, wrote extensively about natural therapies, from his 1838 pamphlet *"Miscellanies of the Gräfenberg Water-Cure"* to comprehensive handbooks published posthumously by his apprentice Theodor Hahn. An early popularizer of natural healing's theory and practice, Rausse claimed that there was only one illness: the disruption or the failure of the body's regulatory apparatus. The "capriciously constructed Genera and Species of illnesses," argued Rausse, "simply do not exist. . . . In pathological types, no individual illness and no sick individual is the same as another, just more or less so."[43] In some individuals, for example, poor digestion might cause sleeplessness. In others, it might lead to fatty deposits in the arteries. These were physical expressions of an underlying regulatory disruption.[44] The healer's job was to identify the link between symptoms and their underlying cause.

Nor was "sickness" necessarily a bad thing. In fact, the symptoms that most doctors mistook for "illness" were actually the body's attempt to heal itself.[45] Just as fever-induced sweating might cleanse the body, or severe headaches might force restfulness on an otherwise overactive patient, the symptoms of regulatory disorder were signs to be read, and warnings to be heeded.[46] Rausse, like Hufeland, claimed that "illness is the deviation from normal metabolic functions."[47] The goal of the healer was always and only to support the body in its efforts to restore regulatory balance.

In much of this, Rausse followed Hufeland, who thought that treating symptoms "[stops] the disease from showing itself outwardly, without paying attention to the remote causes and consequences." In trying to control the physical expression of sickness, the doctor "only destroys the active counteraction of nature, by which it endeavors to remove the real disease: he quenches the fire outwardly, but suffers it to burn more violently within."[48] The use of medications to combat these symptoms introduced additional toxins into the blood stream, digestive tract, etc., thereby retarding the body's efforts to purify itself.[49] Unlike the doctor with his medicine chest and his scalpel, the natural healer sought only "to support the body in its healing endeavor."[50] In this project, Rausse and generations of natural healers who followed him thought that "healthy and easily digestible food, water, clean air, mild warmth, light, electricity, movement, and rest"[51] were the only "natural" therapies.

The natural healer could support patients in restoring balance to their regulatory systems and improving digestion, respiration, and circulation. But the everyday decisions about what to eat or drink, how much to sleep, or whether or not to exercise would ultimately determine how well each individual body functioned. This new attention to the individual's role in preventive health care was one reason that Rausse and other advocates of natural healing actively targeted the reading public with their manuals on health and healing. Patients had to become partners in stopping disease before it started, and to become partners, they needed to be taught about how their bodies really worked. New cultures of popular science and publicity made it easier to reach these audiences.

Beginning around the time that Rausse was writing his *Introduction to Water and Nature Cures* in the 1840s, a new phenomenon was taking shape in German-speaking lands. Educated citizens who had long participated in civic associations were turning to the popular sciences for social and intellectual stimulation.[52] Popular science was both education and entertainment, and the popularity of public demonstrations, exhibitions, and lectures continued to grow well into the twentieth century. The famous International Hygiene Exhibition in Dresden in 1911, for example, attracted more than 5 million visitors.[53]

The popularization of science also shaped the relationship between scientific experts and educated consumers. While popular manuals, open lectures, and public demonstrations all served to celebrate the principles and methods of scientific research—thereby ascribing to experts a kind of privileged social role[54]—they also presumed that science was essentially transparent, and therefore accessible to educated citizens.[55] In principle, popular science ought to have made the relationship between experts and consumers of scientific knowledge more egalitarian. In practice, the situation was more complicated, because the popular literature produced by scientific experts made distinctions between *kinds* of participants—expert and layman, bourgeois and worker, man and woman.[56] This tension was, however, particularly visible in the popular medical literature, where university-trained doctors wrote pamphlets, household handbooks, and instructive brochures designed to educate the public about the mechanics of the body and the logic of illness, at the same time that they warned their patients always to consult with medical experts before taking action.[57]

Rausse, on the other hand, wanted to reclaim knowledge about health and the body from the experts. He believed that, if everyday choices determined the continually shifting relationship between "sickness" and "health," then individuals, not the experts who were called in to treat symptoms, were the key to regulating this relationship. Why, Rausse asked, did so many doctors prescribe medications to treat symptoms rather than the underlying causes of regulatory disruption? Medical men turned to prescriptions rather than to popular education because they had a professional interest in keeping their patients ignorant about how to prevent illness. If the public recognized that "sickness" was the cumulative effect of a lifetime of everyday choices, it would be able to reclaim an authority it had increasingly ceded to doctors. This recognition, though, required a kind of moral courage: while some people "bend only before the force of reason," there were others who would always submit to "the appearance of authority."[58] Rausse told his readers to throw off the shackles of medical elites and submit only to the laws of nature. His call to arms rested on a widely shared belief that medicine's technical language was part of an effort to exclude the lay public from arenas in which it had historically participated.[59] Rausse thought that the doctor's goal should be to "make himself dispensable."[60]

Rausse was critical of the medical doctors who used medications to treat symptoms because he thought that they ignored the role that individuals could play in ensuring their own health. His holistic approach also led him to criticize his old master, Vincenz Prießnitz. Like many others, Rausse was disturbed by reports about the brutality of Prießnitz's use of water—internally and externally—as well as his inattention to diet in the course of the cure.[61] The case described below helps to explain why natural healers increasingly focused their attention not just on the cure, but on prevention and prophylaxis.

The so-called healing crisis was an event that natural healers greeted with cautious optimism because it signaled the body's continuing ability to expel toxic substances. It was also a dangerous time for the patient because, if incorrectly managed, it could lead to the deterioration of a patient's condition and, in the worst cases, death. One patient's vivid description of his own healing crisis while under Prießnitz's care helps to explain why some were critical of Prießnitz.

Dr. Carl Munde came to Gräfenberg in the late 1830s complaining of chronic gout. The first weeks of his residence saw signs of improvement, but at some point, his condition took a dramatic turn for the worse. During the ensuing confinement, the pain became increasingly intolerable and was marked by the appearance of a visible blood clot that caused a "monstrous swelling" of his left hand.[62] High fever with sweats and other liquid emissions followed (he noted, "*alle meine Säfte schienen im Aufruhr zu sein*" [all of my bodily fluids appeared to be in turmoil]), and he had to be continually packed in moist cloths to avoid dehydration. Finally, boils began to appear on his body (he counted no fewer than 54 of them), signaling a healing crisis and the end of his period of confinement.[63]

This "healing crisis" slowly passed, and Munde fell back into the rhythms of Gräfenberg.[64] As chronic pain and fatigue persisted, though, Munde began to think that the cure was almost as bad as the complaint that had brought him to Gräfenberg in the first place. He was particularly critical of the absence of dietary prescriptions. How, he wondered, were patients to purify their bodies if all they were given was fatty meat and heavy sauces?[65] This critical view of hydrotherapies—of their inconsistency and one-sidedness—was becoming widespread, and it led to new thinking about the relationship between health and day-to-day practice.[66] As natural therapies became increasingly comprehensive in their scope, natural healers began to think about how eating and drinking, exercising and recreating might have consequences not just for individual health and well-being, but also for public health and for the life of the nation.[67] In the process, "nature" was reimagined, not just as a model for "the cure" but for healthy living. It was the barely disguised foundation of a protohygienic discourse that imagined healthy living as a total social practice. As part of this shift, we see the term *Wasserheilkunde* replaced with *Naturheilkunde*, an umbrella term that included prescriptions for prevention, lifestyle, and therapy.[68] In attempting to broaden the conception of natural healing, Lorenz Gleich became the first person to systematically define *Naturheilkunde*.

NATURHEILKUNDE: FORMALIZING THE PRINCIPLES AND PRACTICES

The military doctor Lorenz Gleich agreed with Hufeland and Rausse that allopathic doctors confused symptoms with disease and failed to recognize that medicating patients retarded the patients' ability to restore the body's regulatory balance.[69] If allopathic medicine was flawed in its basic assumptions, Gleich thought that water cures like those of Prießnitz were also misguided. Baths, showers, sweat-inducing wraps, drinking water, and spritzes were certainly better than poisoning the body with chemicals. But these practices could not restore the body to a healthy balance if the patient failed to see everyday decisions as the key to health.[70] To combat the one-sidedness of allopathic medicine, but also of water therapies, Gleich proposed a total approach to health and healing that included a rational diet, water, fresh air, sunlight, and exercise.[71]

Gleich first developed this position in an 1850 lecture entitled "On the History of Natural-Healing Practices from Ancient Times until the Present," arguing that the failure to define natural therapies in the first decades of the nineteenth century had stunted their development. Because water therapies played such an important role in natural healing, the public had taken to using terms like "*Wasserheilkunde*" and "hydrotherapy." These descriptions ended up shaping the way that practicing healers thought about their work. It was one reason that they focused on water therapies to the exclusion of other important techniques, including dietary restrictions and exercise regimes.[72]

To combat these problems, Gleich proposed the term *Naturheilkunde* to describe a system that included both health and healing. *Naturheilkunde* would consist of two separate but related parts. The first part, called *Naturdiätetik*, should concern itself with prophylaxis on the basis of "a completely natural lifestyle (*eine vollkommen naturgemäße Lebensweise*) as dictated by the instincts." Eventually, *Naturdiätetik* would cover everything from nutrition to exercise, work and rest, hygiene, sexual activity, and education. As chapter 2 shows, the fact that *Naturdiätetik* could be continually expanded to include new areas of daily life was one of the reasons that natural healing became so successful during the Wilhelmine era.

The second part of Gleich's *Naturheilkunde* was the practice of natural healing, or *Naturheilverfahren*.[73] Natural healers from Prießnitz to Rausse had developed *Naturheilverfahren* more or less systematically over a period of decades, and many of these practices had their origins in medical models that stretched back centuries. Gleich argued, though, that natural healing was fragmented by the myriad healers who developed their therapies without reference to overarching principles. Identifying these principles was an important first step in bringing natural healing to a wider public.

Gleich was not, ultimately, particularly helpful in identifying these principles. In lectures and pamphlets, he reminded healers that nature was a guide for both prevention and treatment, that the body was governed by natural laws, and that healers *and regular people* could identify these laws if they listened to their natural instincts. But he did not tell his audience what it was that nature had to say. And this is because he thought that everyone already knew how to live the natural lifestyle. *Naturheilverfahren* was not about creating something new, but recovering something that had been lost. After all, "so-called primitive peoples know by native instinct what the educated have assembled in books."[74] This may have been interesting advice in the abstract, but it offered little in the way of practical prescriptions. Whatever his success in defining the substance of *Naturheilverfahren*, he did clearly articulate the role that individuals had to play in ensuring their health.

Gleich is best remembered for his efforts to define *Naturheilkunde*, but he claimed that the most important task for natural healers and their supporters was "to educate the public through open lectures."[75] In Gleich's view, "Science is a republic, and in this land . . . there is no dictatorship, no hierarchy, and no compulsion other than the one . . . that governs through truth, reason, and experience."[76] Advocates and adherents of *Naturheilkunde* increasingly recognized that the public had to be educated about the body, and the proliferation of popular guides to health and healing can be seen as an important consequence of this revelation. Treating patients as partners in health was not a casual by-product of *Naturheilkunde*, but a logical effect. After all, "when illnesses are seen not as sicknesses of the organs but rather as pathological configurations, one can combat them only through a very general preventive stance."[77] As doctors and laypersons wrote about health, hygiene, and the advantages of rational lifestyle practices, they brought patients into the process. Gleich and Rausse advocated for an approach to natural healing that was more holistic, more comprehensive, and more inclusive than the therapies advocated by Prießnitz and his contemporaries, but at mid-century, an emerging *Naturheilkunde* was still more preoccupied with healing than with health. The contributions of Theodor Hahn helped to shift the balance toward prevention.

PUBLICITY: *NATURHEILKUNDE* BUILDS NETWORKS

Johannes Rausse was an outspoken advocate for popular education and increased patient participation in hygiene and prevention, but his work might easily have gone unnoticed: he died young, and his contributions to a new model for health and wellness might easily have passed with him. It fell to another to bring his works to a broader public. Theodor Hahn was born on May 19, 1824, in Ludwigsluft in Mecklenburg to an administrator of the municipal grenadiers. Sickly and pock-marked from childhood vaccination, and suffering from asthma, Hahn died of colon cancer in March 1883 after countless doctor visits. He had been apprenticed to an apothecary in his hometown at the age of 17 and gave up his practice in the summer of 1847 to study under Rausse. After completing a cure with Rausse, Hahn remained to assist him in his practice, moving with him in 1848 to the Alexanderbad in Oberfranken. Though their friendship was short, it was a productive one.[78] After Rausse's death in 1848, Hahn edited and published his work, thereby ensuring the continued circulation of his mentor's ideas. Hahn's introduction to *Naturheilkunde* was heavily influenced by the Gräfenberg cure, where hydrotherapies held pride of place. After Rausse's death, though, Hahn increasingly emphasized dietary restrictions, prescribing a fully vegetarian diet as early as 1852.[79] Hahn's emphasis on dietary and lifestyle restrictions is, for a number of reasons, hardly surprising. We know, for example, that vegetarianism was introduced to German-speaking lands by Gustav Struve, the radical republican and Frankfurt parliamentarian,[80] and that Struve visited Gräfenberg while Prießnitz and Rausse were both in residence. Whatever the mechanism for its transmission, Theodor Hahn made a vegetarian diet a central element of his cures in the decades after Rausse's death. Like Rausse, Gleich, and others of their generation, Hahn claimed that "nature" was not just a model for healing, but also a model for living. In Hahn's view, calls to live the natural lifestyle were one thing, but he wanted to explain what this would mean in daily practice. Vegetarianism was central to this project.[81]

In making his case for vegetarianism, he advanced two different but related arguments. First of all, he claimed that the animals to which humans bore the greatest physical resemblance were herbivorous. Monkeys, apes, chimpanzees, and other primates all had vegetables, fruits, and nuts as their primary form of subsistence. While Hahn never cited Darwin or Haeckel, he seems to have tacked some of their central claims—critics described Darwinism as the "*Affenlehre*"—onto natural philosophical arguments about the "origins of species."[82] Natural history was a central element of his physiological arguments. He believed that, like our distant primate cousins, we should eat only those foods intended by nature.

Hahn also tried to make his case in a deductive way. If nature was the model for daily human behavior, then cooked food was, in any of its forms, "unnatural." There was, after all, no such thing as a hot meal in the "state of nature," and there was certainly no natural precedent for the use of exotic spices in the preparation of daily meals.[83] In Hahn's view, it was the failure to eat foods in accordance with "human nature" that was ultimately responsible for sickness. From infancy and early childhood, humans ate foods and consumed drinks that their bodies were not designed to process. It is easy enough to scoff at Hahn's arguments in retrospect, but in a context where meat consumption was dramatically on the rise, his concern begins to make more sense. It was not only the dramatic transformation of dietary habits that motivated Hahn. The relationship between food consumption, ethics, and political economy was, after all, the subject of debate across the continent and into the Americas.[84] Hahn was part of this lively conversation.

Vegetarianism, with historical roots in the late eighteenth-century ascetic Protestant sects in England and Scotland, was always more than simply a dietary regime, and for Hahn it represented a far-ranging social and ethical reform agenda.[85] Hahn likened the dietary and health reform movement of his time to the German reformation:

> Just as 400 years ago at the beginning of the reformation Ulrich von Hutten exclaimed the spirits awake, the sciences flower, it is a joy (*es ist eine Luft*) to be alive, so can we today rejoice in being witnesses to and participants in the battle that has broken free in all areas of science. . . . The struggle is all encompassing, and goes forward simultaneously on the fields of state, social, and legal questions. . . . . But on no other terrain is the battle more stubborn, more intransigent than it is in questions of the body, in the field of the healing sciences.[86]

In the 1850s and 1860s, in the wake of frustrated aspirations for a German nation-state, the importance of diet and a healthy lifestyle became an increasingly central preoccupation in some reform movements that hoped to transform a German society marred by social, political, and economic tribulations of the most diverse sort.[87] Hahn, for example, would argue that "in the dietary question, one finds the key to the social question, though not, as many of the malcontents presently understand it, as a question of political institutions and reforms. . . . What, I ask you, does formal political freedom matter, when physical, spiritual and moral freedom eludes you?"[88] In Hahn's view, individual freedom was the condition for broad social and political transformation. And individual freedom was only possible if one could control one's own body.[89] Hahn was hardly alone in drawing these connections between diverse areas of individual, social, political, and economic life.

Eduard Baltzer (1814–1887) became a vegetarian within months of receiving Hahn's *Die Naturgemäße Diät* in 1866. Delegate to the 1848 Frankfurt Parliament, first president of the Free Religious collective,[90] and founder of the first vegetarian association in Germany in 1867–68,[91] Baltzer believed that in order to transform society, one had first to change oneself. A healthy diet and a natural lifestyle were not, in Baltzer's view, just personal choices: they were the key to a freer and more egalitarian society.[92] Baltzer wrote and lectured on diverse topics, from republicanism and religious freedom to economic inequality and health and hygiene. In his view, all of these issues were tied to one another. The logic of Baltzer's argument went as follows: Man was, by nature, vegetarian. Faced with hunger, though, Man ate meat.[93] All of this led down a slippery slope: "First one must salt the meat, and the salt makes one thirsty. But water no longer satisfies the excited nerves. Then comes the endless row of spices and intoxicating drinks, narcotic pleasures of the most diverse sorts."[94] The desire for luxuries (spices, intoxicating drinks, narcotic pleasures of the most diverse sorts) contributed to the impulse to accumulate wealth. The drive for wealth contributed to economic inequalities. Economic inequalities led to class tensions.[95] For Baltzer, there were direct lines between dietary practices and social organization: unhealthy bodies, like unequal societies, were the result of ignoring the laws of nature. Baltzer had tried political reform in the 1840s. Now, he pressed his agenda on a variety of fronts. One of these was vegetarianism. Like Hahn, Baltzer wrote cookbooks to help interested readers simplify their diets, and to get more in touch with the natural lifestyle. There were recipes for every day of the year.[96]

Many readers will find Baltzer's suggestions naïve—as did many of his contemporaries. In the next chapter, I show how prescriptions for health, hygiene, and social transformation would continue to evolve during the Wilhelmine era. For present purposes, though, I simply want to chart the ways that a body of ideas concerned with therapies was being transformed into a holistic system that addressed everything from water therapies to dietary practices, from healing to health. As natural healers began to focus on health more than healing, they also began to intervene in society in different ways. In the process, nature itself was transformed, from a model for the cure to a guide for everyday living. As I hope to show in the next chapter, this change in the way Germans thought about nature and health had far reaching consequences.

CONCLUSION: "NATURE" TRANSFORMED? FROM HEALING TO HEALTH, 1800–1870

A variety of genealogies could explain why a peasant healer in Austrian Silesia might see the actions of a wounded stag as an appropriate guide for healing a human body (in the first instance, his own). For our purposes, though, it does not really matter which genealogy explains more, or whether there was ever even a stag at all. What matters is that contemporaries persistently told this story, and this story tells us something about how nature was imagined and how it was used in German-speaking lands in the first part of the nineteenth century. Prießnitz, and those who told his story, thought nature was an ordered system that could be deciphered through observation. This is why a stag might offer insights into healing. Animals can only—or so the logic goes—operate according to the laws of nature. For Prießnitz, nature might be a model for healing. But it could not reasonably be imagined as a model for living because that would mean losing *human* nature.

This thinking, and the complex of nature concepts that it held loosely together, shifted in the 1830s and 1840s as Rausse, Hahn, and others began to think about the relationships between natural healing and healthful living. If the principles of nature could be used to heal sick bodies, could they also be leveraged to ensure healthful living? A series of practical questions arose with which natural healers would struggle for decades. "Getting back to nature" or living the "natural lifestyle" was all well and good. But where was "nature," and in what way could the natural world be a model for human behavior? Were all animals natural, or were some more natural than others? These were, increasingly, questions that natural healers, their patients, and their critics had to grapple with.

This does not mean that natural healers themselves were always clear on this point. Hahn, for example, continued to suggest that vegetarianism was "physiological" because our nearest animal relatives were

vegetarian. Hahn was not calling on his readers to return to a prein-
dustrial Eden. His position, and that of many of his contemporaries,
was shot through with contradictions. Nature was an unqualified
good. But only within reason. Neither Hahn nor his contemporaries
imagined that the cities should be torn down, the postal networks dismantled, or the markets shuttered. The contradictions in these kinds
of arguments were possible to ignore in the abstract, but they are pretty obvious when it means telling individuals how, exactly, to live the
natural lifestyle or follow their natural instincts.

Natural healers may have had problems defining what key categories
meant, but one thing was very clear: they hoped to make patients into
partners in health.[97] Rausse, Gleich, Hahn, Baltzer, and others advanced
ideas about nature and the natural lifestyle that were closely tied to this
preventive stance and brought into focus the individual's ability to ensure his or her own well-being. As nature and naturist ideas circulated
in German-speaking lands through self-help manuals, vegetarian cookbooks, sanitaria, and social and ethical reform movements, so too did this
preoccupation with prevention. This was tremendously important because, while natural healers were turning their attention *toward* a preventive medicine that would make doctors "dispensable," mainstream medical
theory was turning *away* from this protohygienic stance, focusing instead
on the localization of illness, the identification of disease categories, and
the isolation of bacteria and viruses.

As we shall see in the next chapter, popular therapies like *Naturheilkunde* developed in a variety of different directions after unification in
1871, and these different trajectories entailed different kinds of social
and cultural beliefs. The idea that nature could be a guide to health
and healing was sometimes a matter of principle, while in other cases it
was a loosely held belief. For some, the belief that nature was a model
for everyday living meant that society needed to be transformed, while
for others, nature only guided individual choices. The story is a complicated one, but one thing is very clear. Naturist thinking saturated
the German experience, particularly during the Wilhelmine period between roughly 1890 and 1918. It is also clear that, for all the political,
social, and cultural differences that inform naturist thinking, there was
broad agreement that nature offered a model for everyday practice, and

that the natural lifestyle was the key to preserving health and preventing illness. Rausse, Hahn, Baltzer, and others wrote about these ideas and helped bring them into focus. In the chapter that follows, we will see the process accelerate dramatically. As naturist thinking saturated the Wilhelmine experience (in self-help books, lectures, retail outlets, sport and bathing facilities, association meetings, reform and policy initiatives), it also introduced the general public to a hygienic discourse focused on prevention and wellness.

CHAPTER TWO

WILHELMINE NATURE
Natural Lifestyle and Practical Politics in the German Life-Reform Movement, 1890–1914

The Wilhelmine era saw the proliferation of popular health and hygiene reform movements that called on Germans to "get back to nature," to live the "natural lifestyle" (*naturgemäße Lebensweise*), and to "celebrate nature." What, though, did this mean? Did "getting back to nature" mean rejecting science and technology, art and culture? Was "nature" an essentially utopian category, and if so, how did this shape the way that contemporaries thought about urban space? Thomas Lekan and Thomas Zeller have shown that "Germany's nature" was always also a cultural artifact.[1] But the very concept of nature has always been profoundly historical, meaning different things at the beginning of the nineteenth century than it did in the 1850s or on the eve of the First World War. By looking at practical politics and consumer culture, this chapter explores the different ways that nature was imagined and understood in the Wilhelmine era. In organizations like the German League for Natural Lifestyle and Therapy Associations (*Deutscher Bund der Vereine für naturgemäße Lebens- und Heilweise*),[2] but also in groups devoted to bathing, gymnastics, vegetarianism, and land reform, Germans from across the social and political spectrum claimed that nature was the key to imagining different and better futures.[3] In some cases, these futures were realized. In others, they have disappeared from historical view.

Historians have long been suspicious of the so-called naturist movements.[4] Citing well-known cultural critics and reactionary ideologues, historians like George Mosse, Fritz Stern, and Klaus Bergmann have taken calls to "get back to nature" as evidence for a widespread "disenchantment with modernity" that would ultimately destabilize Weimar parliamentary politics.[5] More recently, historians who are perhaps influenced by the sociologist Pierre Bourdieu have used what I call a "compensation" model to explain the broad appeal of naturist movements.[6] They suggest that Germans from a variety of class backgrounds "turned to nature" in reaction to the uncomfortable experience of modernization. This tradition has given rise to important work by Michael Hau and Michael Cowan, among others.[7] At least implicitly, though, the compensation argument made so famously by Bourdieu is a teleological one. Here, naturist movements are viewed as both an essentially inadequate response to the logic of the modern and a failure to grasp the realities of an increasingly global capitalist modernity.

Although historians now largely reject the claim that naturist movements laid the foundations for the Nazis and their so-called blood and soil romanticism, the questions today's scholars have been asking remain surprisingly similar to those asked by advocates of the Sonderweg hypothesis decades ago.[8] Was the Life-reform movement (Lebensreformbewegung) progressive or reactionary, practical or utopian? Is land reform (Bodenreform) forward-looking or romantic? Are natural therapies alternative epistemologies or antiscientific populism? While a younger generation of historians has rightly emphasized the progressive elements in naturist movements, that generation has remained susceptible to the lure of familiar, but unhelpful, binaries (modern versus antimodern, progressive versus reactionary).[9] The 2005 collection How Green Were the Nazis? is just one indication that nature remains a powerfully freighted category in the historical imagination.[10]

In the chapter that follows, I try to reframe the problem of "Wilhelmine nature" by distinguishing between different kinds of experience and different ways of imagining the future. First of all, I explore the conceptions of nature presupposed by different programs for social and economic reform, and I contrast these notions with a classically liberal view of nature. Nature figured frequently in Wilhelmine debates about individual health and social reform, and these debates offer important insights into extraparliamentary political culture. In exploring these different and sometimes competing visions, it is not my intention to suggest that nature was either implicitly or necessarily political. Instead, I hope to show some of the ways that nature was used to make social, political, and economic claims. As popular health and hygiene advocacy groups like the German League began increasingly to engage with issues of urban transformation, they also subtly changed the ways that nature was imagined and understood: nature became a tool that could be used to build a better future.

Nature figured so prominently in Wilhelmine popular and political culture not only because of the work of activists from different ideological camps. As we shall see in the second part of the chapter, consumer habits and day-to-day practices played a decisive role in the spread of naturist thinking. To better understand how consumer and lifestyle choices contributed to the circulation of naturist thinking in the Wilhelmine period and beyond, the second part of the chapter looks at Open-Air baths (*Licht-Luftbäder*), which were sites for urban sport and recreation that began to pop up in the 1890s. In the last chapter, we saw Rausse, Gleich, Hahn, and others arguing that nature could be a model not just for the cure, but for everyday living. Open-Air baths—which provided a respite from the pressures of urban living—were seen by their supporters as a way to make nature a part of the urban everyday. In hundreds of these urban oases, but also in serial publications and retail outlets, nature was domesticated for human consumption. Wilhelmine nature was not only a philosophical category deployed to condemn "materialism" or "decadence." Neither was it just a vehicle for progressive social and economic reforms. Wilhelmine nature was, in different hands, something to be enjoyed in sun parks, celebrated in natural healing associations, and achieved through social and economic reform. By exploring these competing visions, I hope to offer an alternative to the frustrating and familiar questions about German modernity.

BUILDING NATURE'S METROPOLIS: THE GERMAN LEAGUE AND LAND REFORM

The German League was founded in 1889 to celebrate nature and natural therapies, to educate the public about health and the body, and to defend the rights of lay healers in Germany's largely unregu-lated medical marketplace.[11] By far the largest health and hygiene ad-vocacy group in Germany, the German League drew its membership from across the confessional divide and the political spectrum.[12] It gave voice to liberals and socialists, social conservatives and sex researchers. Whatever their social or political orientation might have been, though, members of the German League agreed that nature was the key to or-ganizing experience and realizing better futures.[13] If there was broad agreement on that score, it does not follow that social and political dif-ferences were unimportant, particularly when it came to health and the body: it may be true, as one commentator claimed in 1913, that there is no such thing as a "social democratic intestine, nor a conservative liver or kidney." But there certainly have been Social Democratic health care models, just as there have been Conservative and National Lib-eral ones.[14] These different ways of thinking about health and hygiene closely mirrored the ways that group members thought about other is-sues, like wages, tax policy, public housing, and welfare institutions. In the pages that follow, I want to highlight some of these different and often competing visions.

Nature: Liberal Perspectives

Some in the natural healing movement harnessed "Wilhelmine na-ture" to a classically liberal narrative that stressed education, individual responsibility, self-help, and personal choice. Members of the Associa-tion for Healthcare and Nonmedicinal Healing Neustadt-Reudnitz in Leipzig (*Verein für Gesundheitspflege und arzneilose Heilweise*) claimed, for example, that their organization hoped to "spread knowledge of natural lifestyles and healing to its members," paying particular atten-tion to the "physical and moral education" of the children.[15] Although the Neustadt-Reudnitz association was just one of the 638 local chap-ters making up the German League in 1907, their mission, variously phrased, was written into the charter of many associations.[16] The natural healing association in the Gohlis district of Leipzig had a different take on the classically liberal story, linking individual choice with the fate of the nation. Writing to the Leipzig city council in 1909, they claimed, "it is the foremost duty of any person who hopes to successfully serve his age (*Zeitalter erfolgreich dienen*) to keep his body healthy and free from unnatural influences."[17] Education, individual responsibility, and choice were, in this view, the key to personal well-being and the health of the nation.

Magnus Hirschfeld also focused on the relationship between the individual and the state, claiming that "those who assume that well-being depends exclusively, or even primarily, on the state commit a serious error."[18] He cited approvingly the words of the poet Maurice Reinhold von Stein, who wrote, "It is not just a reform of state and society that is necessary, but also a reform of lifestyle and of character.... Without first fighting for temperance, I would not be able to suppress the fear that a shorter working day and higher pay would also result in a greater frequency of public houses."[19] Magnus Hirschfeld is best known as a sexologist and advocate for the decriminalization of homosexuality, but in the 1890s he was also an important voice in the German League. In "Self-Help or State-Aid" and in other pieces published in *Nature's Doctor*, Hirschfeld, like members of the Leipzig Gohlis association, took aim at health and hygiene reformers who thought that state action was the key to improving health outcomes.[20]

Nature: Left-Liberal and Socialist Perspectives

General appeals to the healing power of nature—along with calls to live right—were one thing. But in the high era of urbanization, between roughly 1880 and 1910, some Life-reformers began increasingly to wonder how they were supposed to "live naturally," "get back to nature," and listen to their "natural instincts."[21] Between 1871 and 1914, for example, Berlin grew 249 percent, from about 800,000 to more than 2 million, and while Berlin was Germany's largest city, its growth was still relatively slow. Leipzig, for example, grew 585 percent during the same period, Hamburg 346 percent, and Cologne 496 percent.[22] Some in the natural healing movement continued to call on Germans to transform their own bodies by "getting back to nature." They continued to educate their members about preventive practice and to advocate the "natural lifestyle." But when nutritionists at the office of public health determined that a working-class family of four could expect to spend roughly 70 percent of their income for a subsistence diet at a time when these families made up nearly 75 percent of the population of Prussia, the case that everyone should "get back to nature" became increasingly difficult to swallow.[23] And when Nobel Prize-winning bacteriologist Robert Koch argued that inadequate housing was the "incubator" of tuberculosis, it was hard to ignore the indexical ties between health and wealth.[24] The classically liberal story about self-help, individual responsibility, lifestyle, and choice was under serious pressure, not just from health and hygiene experts, but also from the growing working-class voting public. With Social Democrats making gains at the municipal and national levels, health and hygiene reform took on a new urgency.[25]

Aware of shifts within the public health community, and motivated by the changing face of German cities, some within the natural healing movement began to demand practical initiatives and public health solutions to the problems of the urban experience. As Alfred Knoll, a Social Democrat and member of the German League, wrote in an editorial published in *Nature's Doctor* (*Naturarzt*), it was time to move beyond the "well-known cookbook formula" that tells readers to eat prescribed foods and drink particular drinks, to take the cure at one facility, and to visit another for daily sport and fitness activities. For many Germans struggling to put food on the table and roofs over their heads, this advice was totally beside the point. For these Germans, the "cookbook formula" offered by popular health and hygiene movements like the German League mostly raised questions. For Knoll, the most important of these questions was not which ingredient to take when following a recipe for healthy living. The question was rather "how do I 'take' it if I do not steal it?"[26] In pieces with titles like "The Natural Healing Movement and the Right of Assembly" and "The Natural Healing Movement and Food Taxes," Knoll was just one of many voices calling for a more active engagement with the policy issues that defined public health, from urban green space and housing reform, to wage and tax issues.[27] Wilhelmine nature, it turns out, was as easily articulated in Social Democratic or Left-Liberal language as it was open to classically liberal interpretations.[28] In part because of this polyvocal quality, categories like "modern," "antimodern," and "reactionary" fail to adequately account for the complexity of Wilhelmine nature.

The growing concern with social and economic issues did not mean that nature disappeared from the conceptual field, and in the 1890s and early 1900s, left-leaning members of naturist movements like the German League continued to argue that the natural lifestyle was one important key to ensuring health and happiness. As Dr. Ernst Wilms, the Lord Mayor of Posen from 1903–1918, noted, there was clear evidence of the causal relationship between "physical and psychic health, and the proximity to nature." He argued that green space was without question "a counterweight to the negative health consequences of the city."[29] We also know from contemporary ethnographic studies by Adolf Levenstein and Paul Göhre that workers were as anxious to take care of their bodies, spend time in parks and forests, breathe clean air, and have adequate housing as were other Germans.[30] One of Levenstein's informants, a 22-year-old weaver, said that after spending the workweek in rooms with "damp, dusty, foul-smelling air," he was "happy . . . to explore the outdoors and nature."[31] Another turned to the classics to make his point: "I think of Goethe's words, 'Oh how glorious is nature, how the sun shines and the meadows laugh.'"[32] Nature, in short, was a central category not just for classically liberal voices in the German League, but also for Social Democrats and Left-Liberals. If nature and the natural lifestyle remained a key part of this reform culture, though, reformers argued that this had to be balanced with the particular challenges posed by the changing urban experience. In the first decades of the twentieth century, the German League increasingly turned its attention to the practical work of transforming German cities, proceeding from an idea of nature that was distinct from the classically liberal version. Building on the personal and institutional networks that crisscrossed the Life-reform movement, the German League formed some surprising alliances in the process. Collaboration with the League of Land Reformers is just one example of how different Life-reformers used nature to create spaces of mutual interest.

Nature, Land Reform, Life-reform

Land reform (*Bodenreform*) may not seem an obvious outlet for the energies of the natural healing movement, though at least three of the editors at *Nature's Doctor* between 1894 and 1925 held advisory positions in the national association.[33] But as studies multiplied during the 1890s and early 1900s linking public health to problems like land speculation, rising ground rents, housing shortages, and urban overcrowding, important figures in the German League and from across the Life-reform movement increasingly made the case that land reform was also public health reform. In the pages of *Nature's Doctor*, for example, the novelist and feminist activist Anna Pappritz argued that key public health problems—from tuberculosis to prostitution—were tied to urban poverty and overcrowding. While there was a 10.3 percent incidence of tuberculosis-related deaths in single-family apartments with six or more rooms where one household member was infected, the figure jumped to 42.2 percent in shared two-room apartments.[34] The Bauhaus architect Peter Behrens also took the broad view, telling an audience in 1915 that, if they ever hoped to solve the problems facing German cities—the overflowing hospitals and the living quarters shared by as many as ten people—they would have first to solve the "land question" (*Bodenfrage*).[35] For Pappritz as for other reformers, it was not a question of "nature" *or* social and economic reform. The "natural lifestyle" was, instead, something to be *achieved* through systemic social and economic reform. This was a case that land reformers had been making since the early 1890s.

Land reformers like Adolf Damaschke and Friedrich Naumann claimed that Germany's demographic revolution was placing continually expanding demand-side pressure on a fixed commodity. As long as industrial production continued to grow, and as long as workers continued to move to cities to find work, demand for housing would exceed supply.[36] Land-reform advocate W. Heinrich complained, for example, that real estate owners and landlords were making vast sums without actually having to do any real work. Steadily rising rents resulted not from the work of land speculators but from "the expansion of the city, which makes outlying areas more central through the construction of gas and water lines, trams and omnibuses, churches and schools."[37] Cities built infrastructure, industry provided jobs, workers offered their labor, and real estate dealers made the profits. In Heinrich's view, this was unsustainable from both social and public health perspectives. Citing data generated by Heinrich Herkner, professor

at the University of Berlin, Heinrich pointed out that many German
workers were spending more than 30 percent of their wages on rent,
with the result that mothers and children were often forced into the
labor market, and families were living in cramped, unhygienic apartments. This was, Heinrich went on to say, "particularly dangerous for
the children. . . . In epidemics, houses with tightly packed and overcrowded apartments have the highest mortality rates." In Heinrich's
view, land reform was the key to solving the related problems of urban
overcrowding and epidemic disease.[38]

To hedge against the uncontrolled rise in ground rents, land reformers proposed, among other things, incremental taxes on capital gains,
increased municipal ownership of lands outside of expanding city centers, and a more rational planning of urban growth through advisory
boards and popular input.[39] Key voices in the German League gave
their strong endorsement to these proposals. In a review of Damaschke's National Economy in 1910, for example, founding member of
the German League Wilhelm Siegert told Nature's Doctor readers that
"no association library should be without it." He went on to argue that,
"without land reform, healthy housing . . . is unthinkable. For this reason we followers of the natural healing movement must fully engage
with these questions."[40] This was a message that resonated far beyond
the Life-reform movement. As Lord Mayor Heinrich von Wagner of
Ulm said in a speech celebrating Damaschke's accomplishments, "thousands of town leaders and city councillors"[41] believed that land reform
was the key to improving public health.

At first, it may not be easy to see what all of this had to do with
nature, the natural lifestyle, and getting back to nature. In the context
of changing urban landscapes and evolving health and hygiene sciences,
though, many in the Life-reform movement thought that social and
economic reform was the necessary condition for the natural lifestyle,
the key to transforming the urban experience. As member of the German League's executive committee Paul Schirrmeister put it, "Tuberculosis, sexually transmitted diseases and nervous dissipation. . . are ills of
the metropolis, with its barracks-living and overcrowded apartments,
the deprivation of city-dwellers of air, light, room, and of natural stimu-
lae more generally."[42] Calls to get back to nature and to live more natu-

ral lives were all well and good, but they could only be realized when systematic reforms had been put in place. Schirrmeister, for his part, advocated the massive de-scaling of urban centers along lines proposed by Garden-city pioneers Silvio Gessells and Ebenzer Howard. His proposals were simple: "fresh clean air, clean healthy drinking and bathing water, safe and speedy removal of sewage."[43] Like other Garden-city advocates, Schirrmeister ultimately hoped to establish a "lasting connection of all segments of the population, but particularly the young, with *authentic Nature.*"[44]

Schirrmeister's call for more green space and improved ventilation in housing appears quite reasonable in retrospect, but historians have sometimes viewed this kind of culture critique as irrational, antimodern, and even anti-Semitic. The incendiary language that Life-reformers sometimes used—the "Metropolis as Moloch" is a phrase made familiar by Clemens Zimmerman and Jürgen Reulecke in their collection of the same title—goes some way in explaining historians' concern.[45] But Schirrmeister's was not a blanket criticism of cities as such. His was a critique of German cities as they existed in the first decade of the twentieth century, with too many people in too little space, too many factories and not enough parks. Schirrmeister may have been outspoken in his criticism of the metropolis, but his concerns were widespread. As he pointed out, the natural healing movement had made its largest gains in membership in urban areas, "where an ever stronger . . . longing for hygiene reform is felt."[46] Schirrmeister's was not a call to recreate a utopian past, but rather a vision for building a better future. Historian Edward Ross Dickinson has suggested in a recent review article that these imagined futures were hardly isolated, nor were they confined to the fringes.[47] Naturist movements were central to this reform milieu.

I do not want to spend too much time here tracing out the personal and institutional networks that helped to shape the broad Wilhelmine reform agenda, but it is worth noting, at least briefly, how extraordinarily dense this milieu really was. Adolf Damaschke, as we know, edited *Nature's Doctor* before leaving to lead the League of Land Reformers and the Garden-city Movement;[48] feminist activist Anna Pappritz regularly commented on the relationship between housing and public health;[49] and Franz Schönenberger, who edited *Nature's*

meetings in associational meeting-houses were important ways not just of maintaining group solidarity, but also of relaxing and having fun. At a time when cities were rapidly growing, and migration was becoming increasingly common, local associations created ways of knowing places that would otherwise have eluded many Germans in changing urban environments. To newly arrived members, they transformed unfamiliar socialscapes into ones inhabited by like-minded individuals. To long-time residents of rapidly changing towns and cities, they offered ways of understanding changing environments. Associations allowed members to draw on the knowledge and experiences of other members, who included people they might otherwise never encounter.

One practical consequence of this intimacy can be seen in the demographic makeup and ideological orientation of individual associations. Unlike the German League as a whole, which drew its membership from across the demographic spectrum, local associations could be fairly homogeneous in their composition. In cities like Leipzig, Berlin, and Dresden—but also in smaller cities like Chemnitz, Zwickau, or Oldenburg—individuals could choose between numerous natural healing associations. In some cases, these choices were dictated by proximity or by personal connections. Individuals could, for example, choose to join the associations closest to their homes, or they might be invited to join by a friend or work colleague. In other cases, the decision to join one association rather than another might be based on the ideological priorities expressed by group members in lectures or pamphlets. In practice, this meant that particular associations were often relatively homogenous in demographic and/or ideological terms, despite the fact that the German League as a whole retained its diversity.

It is difficult to ascertain why individuals chose to join the associations that they did. But the consequences of these choices are apparent in the decisions taken by local associations, the initiatives these local chapters pursued, and the conflicts that sometimes arose within group meetings. An annual report from the Association for Natural Health Care in Leipzig-Kleinzschocher (*Verein für naturgemäße Gesundheitspflege—Leipzig Kleinzschocher*), for example, tells us that, in 1900, only nine of twenty-six association meetings were pedagogical in content. The high percentage of social events dotting the annual calendar—

seasonal celebrations, children's festivals, family outings, and other purely social engagements, for example—suggests that members of the Kleinzschocher group were more interested in spending time with one another, engaging in sports and socializing than they were in hearing lectures about personal choice, responsibility, health, and the body. This interpretation finds further support from a detail in the same report, where the authors noted that, while bathing utensils were almost constantly on loan to association members, the same could not be said of the association's library holdings.[58] This was a fairly weak showing for an organization whose mission was to bring "light and enlightenment about generally accessible health care and therapy."[59]

In comparison, one might cite the pedagogical efforts of the Natural Healing Association Leipzig East (*Naturheilverein Leipzig-Ost*), where the membership fee entitled members to visit educational lectures held on each alternating Friday. Membership included a subscription to *Nature's Doctor*; access to the association's library and to bathing utensils (for example, foot and "sitz" baths); and, on lecture evenings, free natural medical advice.[60] In the natural healing movement, institutional mechanisms and federal principle allowed members room to build communities and pursue their own interests without the threat of political or ideological conflict.[61] Nature, despite the many different things that it meant to different members, was a value, an ideal, and a goal for all natural healing associations, whatever their demographic or ideological makeup.

If classical and left-liberal narratives were able to co-exist, though, this did not ultimately resolve underlying differences, and increasingly, left-liberal and socialist concerns defined the public face of the natural healing movement. This preoccupation with a reform agenda is visible in a whole range of popular health and hygiene publications, from *People's Health* (*Volksgesundheit*) and *The New Healing Art* (*Neue Heilkunst*) to *Reform Journal* (*Reformblätter*), and it can be seen in the German League's collaboration with organizations from across the Life-reform movement. It can be seen in efforts to protect Berlin's Grünewald from urban expansion, a decade-long effort that saw the proliferation of action committees, advisory councils, petitions, and plans, all of which were designed to affect local decision-making about how land was used.[62]

Nor were these "marginal" or "fringe" projects. As an English observer noted with surprise in 1904, German towns held more than three times the amount of public land in trust as did cities in his home country. Much of this land was devoted to parks and other green space, a fact he attributed in part to land reform initiatives.[63]

The German League was not, of course, the sole driver of this reformist impulse. Efforts to build health and hygiene standards into housing policy regularly found their way onto the parliamentary floor, and elite organizations played an important role in keeping legislative attention on these kinds of issues.[64] If organizations like the Association for Public Health Care (*Verein für Öffentliche Gesundheitspflege*) represented an important arena for policy debate, popular groups like the German League, the Friends of Nature, and the League of Land Reformers played a different role. Through lectures, petitions, and other popular initiatives, they helped to ensure the broad circulation of "naturist" thinking and draw the public into a conversation about public health and hygiene. For their part, the German League joined the League of Land Reformers as a corporate member in 1908, with one of the German League's founding members claiming that

> the shortage of housing in the big cities and industrial regions will end only when the state and local precincts engage in a broad housing politics. [We should demand] the greatest possible expansion of the communal land as a counter weight to unhealthy land speculation. Our association should support with all our power endeavors with the goal of healthier housing.[65]

Land reform is just one example of an expanded agenda that saw the transformation of German cities as the condition for the "natural lifestyle." In this context, transforming the body social was perceived as a step toward creating natural bodies.

The widespread agreement among members of the German League and in the broader Life-reform movement that nature was an ideal to be celebrated—and that it was a vehicle for the improvement of individual bodies and the amelioration of social circumstances—created a possibility for collaboration in the face of political difference.

This collaborative mood had real consequences. The whole movement might have been a historical footnote, just one among the hundreds of other reform initiatives in the Wilhelmine landscape, but it amounted to something more: through consumer culture, fitness, sport and leisure practices, nature became a part of urban life *not just for those committed followers of natural healing* and not just for health and hygiene reformers. This helps to explain the reception not only of natural therapies, as we will see in subsequent chapters, but also of a broader set of naturist ideas.

DOMESTICATING NATURE: OPEN-AIR BATHS AND THE URBAN EXPERIENCE

It is easy enough to assume that the vogue for "getting back to nature" had something to do with the tremendously influential Wilhelmine celebrities who "took the cure" or claimed to live their lives according to the dictates of nature.[66] Wilhelm II and the Grand Duchess Alexandrine were both believers,[67] as was Konrad Haenisch who, in 1918/19 became the first Social Democratic Minister of Culture. "Nature apostles" like Gusto Gräser, Wilhelm Dieffenbach, and Hugo Höppener attracted attention not only from literary types from Thomas Mann and Gerhardt Hauptmann to Hermann Hesse, but also from the sociologist Max Weber and scientists like Albert Einstein.[68] Ultimately, though, this transformation had less to do with the celebrity intellectuals, politicians, and princely figures who took "the cure" than it did with the new kinds of consumer culture, communication, and publicity.[69]

Created to provide sites for healthy recreation and sport in increasingly densely populated urban centers, Open-Air baths were semiprivate parks in which men and women could walk, practice healing gymnastics, run and take the fresh air, sunbathe in secluded huts, and swim in the nude or in minimal dress.[70] The widespread belief in the salutary effects of fresh air, clean water, and comfortable clothing—common in a variety of reform movements, from clothing reform to body culture—helps to explain the popularity of the Open-Air baths. Claiming that the naked body was neither shameful nor inherently sexual, clothing reformers, body culture advocates, and natural healers all pointed to the health and hygiene benefits of nudity.[71] Best-selling author Adolf Just, who ran a natural healing sanatorium in the Harz, told his readers to "strip the body now and again, and walk about naked . . . in the open air or in a wood,"[72] and many doctors agreed that the Open-Air baths were useful tools in fighting conditions from neurasthenia to tuberculosis.[73] Dr. Georg Liebe of the Sanatorium Waldhof-Elgershausen, for example, told readers of the medical reform publication *Journal for Physical and Dietary Therapy* (*Zeitschrift für physikalische-diätetische Therapie*) that the therapeutic benefits of the Open-Air baths had been proven "in theory and praxis,"[74] and by 1919, the dean of the medical faculty at the University of Berlin was able to tell a parliamentary commission that "no doctor leaves the university . . . without having had the opportunity to study [these] therapies."[75]

These parks turned out to be a shockingly popular innovation: while Franz Kafka kept his underpants on when taking the cure at one such facility, it was sufficiently mainstream for him to have visited.[76] Eric Mühsam and Hermann Hesse also went, as did millions of others in various states of undress.[77] International observers were quick to recognize the importance of this new approach to health and hygiene. One American observer told readers of the *American Monthly Review* that the Open-Air bath "stands for *a new method of returning to nature*."[78] William Paul Gerhard, a civil engineer and member of the American Public Health Association, also commented on this innovation, telling his readers that, beginning in the 1890s, "a general movement [for Open-Air baths] has . . . spread rapidly through Germany . . . largely at the instigation of the *Societies for Natural Methods of Healing and Living*."[79] By 1912, there were more than 380 such baths owned and operated by natural healing associations across Germany. They had quickly become important sites of a natural sociability and health-oriented recreation. Why, though, did Germans need a "new method of returning to nature" in the first place?

Sunbathing can happen anywhere, but the innovation of the Open-Air bath was the enclosure of spaces, the introduction of gender-specific areas, changing and washing rooms, exercise facilities, and the provision of adequate shade and water.[80] These innovations made it possible to exercise, sunbathe, relax, and socialize—either in the nude or in bathing costumes—without *publicly* transgressing those norms that dictated modesty and that governed the interaction between different sexes and age groups. By 1900, the health benefits of "returning to nature" were widely recognized, and fresh air, sunlight, physical exercise in parks—as well as stripping off layers of heavy clothes and constraining corsets—were all seen as part of this "return." As the well-known lifestyle entrepreneur Arnold Rikli put it, "The goal of the atmospheric cure" was not to transform bathers into "nature-people" or "force them back to the wild." Rather, these baths were intended, "to accustom civilized people . . . with the outdoors."[81] From culturally conceived notions of appropriate gender relations to design and maintenance decisions about ideal natural aesthetics, Open-Air baths expressed key *cultural* assumptions held by advocates and adherents of the natural lifestyle. In the Open-Air baths, health-conscious individuals found an intermediate space between overcrowded cities and "the wild." They were able to be consumers of a self-consciously domesticated version of nature.

It was not only body-culture activists or the committed followers of the natural lifestyle who found their way into these parks, and at times the traffic could be quite extraordinary. A Leipzig city councilman estimated that, in the summer season, between 800 and 1,000 residents passed through facilities owned by the natural healing association Leipzig-West *each day*.[82] Even by a conservative estimate, one that takes into account the unpredictable German summer, the Leipzig-West facilities managed some 70,000 visitors per season. And there were hundreds of similar baths across Germany. As early as 1900, some municipalities were providing financial assistance to natural healing associations to help maintain bathing and sport facilities. One memorandum cited the health of working class children, who were particularly affected by issues of urban poverty, as a particular reason to ensure that Open-Air baths continued to be a low-cost option for rest and relaxation.[83] This focus on public health would become even more pronounced during the First World War and in its immediate aftermath.

Given the numbers of people passing through these kinds of facilities each day, it is not surprising that the Open-Air baths sometimes raised concerns within the community. In July 1899, for example, the German Women's Association for the Advancement of Morality (*Deutscher Frauenverein für die Hebung der Sittlichkeit—DFVHS*) petitioned the Saxon Ministry of the Interior to look into some questionable goings-on at the natural healing sanitarium and bathing facilities run by Pastor Emmanuel Felke. Members of the *DFVHS* were particularly concerned that the bathing facilities failed to enforce strict gender separation. This laxity in enforcing the rules of propriety might not have been a problem, except for the fact that guests were encouraged to sunbathe "without bathing trunks or bathing dresses."[84] The authors of the petition cited anonymous testimony claiming that women were sometimes "forbidden from wearing bathing costumes," and if they tried to do so, "were . . . *taunted*," presumably by men from across the fence.[85] Children were also exposed to moral danger. While there was no mention of young girls using the facilities, boys were allowed to roam free, and Felke's nine-year-old son was reported to do so naked.[86]

Concerns expressed in the *DFVHS* petition set off a flurry of correspondence, with letters passing between the offices of the Ministry of Culture, the Ministry of the Interior, local administrators and, because of Felke's religious affiliation, the Royal Consistory (*Königliche Konsistorium*). A memorandum from the Ministry of the Interior to the Ministry of Culture, for example, called the situation "extraordinary, from a moral point of view," and asked for a full report.[87] In response, the Ministry of Culture called on the High Consistory (*Oberkirchenrat*) to conduct a thorough investigation, noting that Felke's actions could have potentially damaging consequences for "church interests."[88] Perhaps most interesting was the line taken by the consistory, which simultaneously defended Pastor Felke to the government and wrote to Felke cautioning him about any appearance of impropriety. "You are," they reminded Felke, "first and foremost a clergyman, and as such must carefully avoid anything that could harm the diocese."[89] In response to concerns expressed by church authorities, construction began on fences that would better separate the men's and women's parts of the baths. In May, local administrators noted with satisfaction that construction had been completed. Appropriate boundaries had been re-established.

This example may seem like a quirky episode, and in a sense, it is. Yet it also captures broader assumptions about the Open-Air baths, the "natural lifestyle," and "getting back to nature." While the women of the DFVHS may have been scandalized by the familiar way in which naked men spoke with scantily clad young women, they did not reject the principles that organized Felke's bathing facilities. "No one," they wrote, "would object to a respectable healing facility."[90] For members of the DFVHS, the problem was not "getting back to nature," the celebration of "natural lifestyle," or even nudism per se—though the latter did raise concerns.[91] What the authors of the petition wanted the authorities to address was the perceived breakdown of gender boundaries and the failure to police cultural norms.[92] Actors on both sides of the fence recognized that getting back to nature was a profoundly cultural practice. Getting back to nature and leading a natural lifestyle were ways of organizing the urban everyday. This is an interpretation borne out by evidence from a variety of sources, all of which suggest the extraordinary extent to which naturist ideas saturated the Wilhelmine experience.

We know, for example, that a flourishing association culture celebrating nature and the natural lifestyle allowed group members, their families, and their guests to attend lectures and social evenings as well as seasonal festivals and weekend expeditions. The associations gave members access to lending libraries and association facilities like sunbaths and sport-parks, and the German League provides an important lens into this world.[93] With approximately 150,000 members in 890 local associations across Germany on the eve of the First World War, the German League was by far the largest health and hygiene advocacy group in the country.[94] According to one contemporary estimate, the local associations that made up the German League offered some 10,000 lectures in 1900.[95] In the case of well-known lecturers like Reinhold Gerling, who edited Nature's Doctor from 1896 to 1906, audiences regularly swelled into the thousands.[96]

These numbers tell only part of the story because the German League was also part of a network of issue-oriented reform movements—what contemporaries called the Life-reform (Lebensreform) movement—that shared institutional resources, and often overlapped in their personnel.[97] According to the Brockhaus dictionary, Life-reform was a complex of movements that had as their common goal the reform of "lifestyle, particularly in the areas of nutrition, clothing, housing, and healthcare."[98] These reform associations began, in the 1890s, to coalesce in a network that shared members, objectives, and sometimes resources.[99] Work done by Florentine Fritzen suggests that, at its peak in 1913/14, the Life-reform network may have counted as many as 4 million people in its ranks.[100]

The vastly expanded corpus of natural healing manuals also played a part in educating middle- and working-class publics about the natural lifestyle. Dozens, even hundreds of these works appeared annually, some of them published by tiny printers, others turning into international bestsellers. In the case of F. E. Bilz's *The New Natural Healing Method* (*Das Neue Naturheilverfahren*), first published in 1888, the success was simply astonishing.[101] In 1894, *The New Natural Healing* sold 200,000 copies. In 1895, it sold 250,000. In 1900, Bilz's book celebrated the publication of its 100th edition. It would eventually be translated into twelve languages and sell more than 3,500,000 copies. New consumer products and retail outlets also had a role to play. In the 1890s and early 1900s, retail outlets selling "natural" and "reform" products were increasingly to be found in most German cities, particularly in the "Hanseatic North, the Ruhr region, the Rheinland, greater Berlin, Saxony, Thuringia and Hesse."[102] If these were too far away for easy access, businesses like the Carl Braun mail-order catalog (*Versandhaus*) made it possible to purchase everything that one needed—from muesli and "reform butter" (margarine) to hygiene and clothing items—to live the natural lifestyle. In the hands of lifestyle entrepreneurs, natural healers, and organizations like the German League, nature was marketed for human consumption.

In the process of getting back to nature, patrons of the Open-Air baths took trams, rode bicycles, paid entrance fees, and joined voluntary associations. In their efforts to live more naturally, they helped Sebastian Kneipp sell hundreds of thousands of volumes (his *My Nature Cure* is still in print) and *Nature's Doctor* reach a circulation of nearly 160,000. They also patronized the 200 vegetarian restaurants in Germany and spent millions on products sold in retail outlets and mail-order catalogs like Carl Braun's.[103] Consumer culture was an important vehicle for the spread of naturist ideas: through self-help manuals, lectures, bathing facilities, and retail outlets, "nature" helped to shape a language known even to those who had little interest in the "natural lifestyle" or the Life-reform project. Even measured in crudest terms that focus on access and exposure to reform products, sites for natural recreation, and ideas about the natural lifestyle, nature was increasingly a part of the every-man's everyday—a possibility for fashioning daily practice, imagining possible futures, eating and drinking, socializing, and staying healthy.[104] This helps us to understand why allegedly marginal associations were able to influence policy decisions, public health practices, and even, as we shall see in the following chapters, the practice of medicine and the production of knowledge.

CONCLUSION

Nature saturated the Wilhelmine experience. It was domesticated in Open-Air baths, sold in retail outlets, and consumed at the breakfast table. It circulated in lectures about hygiene and fitness, and in seri-als and self-help manuals that reached millions. Natural healers and lifestyle entrepreneurs preached the gospel of nature in sanatoria and advertisements. Activists demanded more green space and healthier housing in petitions and town-hall meetings. Even those suspicious of the naturist lifestyle could not ignore it. Hauptmann and Mann both wrote well-known novels with "nature apostles" in mind. The women of the DFVHS wanted the government to do a better job regulating the Open-Air baths. In parliament, one speaker made reference on the parliamentary floor to the lifestyle entrepreneur from Saxony F. E. Bilz and expected colleagues from Bavaria and the Ruhr region to recognize the name (and it appears they did).

Nature was ubiquitous in Wilhelmine conversations about lifestyle, choice, and policy reform, and this had demonstrable effects. Chairs for natural therapies were mandated for all German universities in the in-terwar period, and healthy, natural housing was elevated from a munici-pal concern to a fundamental human right by the Weimar constitution. If nature and naturist thinking saturated the Wilhelmine experience, though, they also meant different things to different people. Whether it was experienced in consumer practice, celebrated in classically liberal language, or achieved through social and economic reform, though, nature was a way of articulating possible futures. Young-sun Hong has rightly argued that the German experience was "[n]either singular nor alternative."[105] In part through the natural healing movement, in part through new consumer cultures and publicity networks, nature became a part of the urban everyday. In the process, it became a way not just for fashioning daily practices but also for planning cities, organizing leisure, and petitioning elected officials.[106] The vision of a holistic health system articulated by Rausse and others in the middle of the nineteenth century had been transformed into something far more than that.

⟨⌒⟩⟨⌒⟩

CHAPTER THREE

CONTESTING THE MEDICAL MARKETPLACE

Politics, Publicity, and Scientific Progress, 1869–1910

In 1869, when the Berlin Medical Association proposed a rider to pending trade legislation lifting all barriers to entry into the medical marketplace, medicine became one of the "Free Professions" open to all persons, regardless of gender, confession, age, education, or accreditation.[1] Passage of this landmark legislation helped to create an extraordinarily unregulated market for medical care in Germany, one that was unique in the European world.[2] At first, doctors saw in the trade act welcome relief from the many duties that, for almost six decades, had come with medical licensing.[3] Chief among these was the so-called "compulsion to provide care," which made the refusal to provide medical services a civil offense.[4] In calling for the incorporation of medicine as one of the free professions, the Berlin Medical Association was not knowingly advocating a more competitive medical marketplace: the rider was part of a more cynical effort to free doctors from a variety of professional obligations, including the "compulsion to provide care."[5]

The consequences of deregulating medical practice in Germany were not immediately clear. After all, doctors had long worked alongside surgeons, apothecaries, midwives, teachers, priests, and other nonlicensed healers, with different practitioners offering services to different kinds of cure-seekers. This was a medical marketplace governed by informal rules, and as Mary Lindemann, Roy Porter, and others have shown, these rules depended in part on a division of therapeutic labor.[6] While the 1869 trade legislation changed the legal framework organizing the relationship between licensed doctors and nonlicensed healers, the *de facto* division of labor did not immediately disappear.[7] However, the situation would change dramatically over the next three decades.

Changes in the relationships between licensed doctors and "other healers" were conditioned by a range of factors, from the creation of a national insurance scheme beginning in 1883, to an increasingly difficult job market for young doctors.[8] The marketplace was also changing in important ways. Beginning in the 1880s, nonlicensed healers increasingly used new media and retail outlets, advocacy groups, associational networks, and other entrepreneurial tactics to broadcast their own therapeutic innovations and create new demand for their services. As nonlicensed healers targeted a more and more diverse audience, as they transgressed the informal rules governing the medical marketplace and encroached upon the traditional client base of licensed doctors, they contributed to a breakdown of the medico-therapeutic division of labor. This process drew doctors, first slowly, then more rapidly, into a competitive relationship with "other healers." In part because of these new, more competitive dynamics, doctors' attitudes toward their nonlicensed colleagues underwent a major shift.[9]

Faced with new and potentially threatening market forces, doctors began to call for the reinstatement of regulatory protections on the professional practice of medicine, and by the late 1890s, German medical associations were actively mobilizing to control the spread of what they called "quackery." They claimed that swindlers and charlatans were seducing the masses with potions and elixirs, and that uneducated laypeople were dangerously susceptible to promises by unscrupulous fakes. In many cases, medical associations were joined in their crusade by bureaucrats, police superintendents, university professors, and other educated elites, and these defensive alliances are important in understanding the asymmetries that organized the medical landscape. This mobilization of the "official" medical community is an important aspect of the present story. Medical lobbyists tried to marginalize other healers by framing the debate between medical epistemologies in the language of class hierarchies: they tried to convince the public that only the uneducated masses would be foolish enough to prefer "other healers" to university-trained doctors. Historians have done excellent work recovering the rich medical landscapes represented by nonconventional healing traditions, but too often scholarship has taken at face value the Wilhelmine medical lobby's self-serving map of the medical marketplace.

As I show in this chapter, the defensive alliance between medical men and some educated elites is only part of the story. Contrary to what contemporary critics of "quackery" would have us believe, attitudes toward nonlicensed healers did not break down along class lines, nor did an individual's level of education necessarily dictate his or her perception of a free medical marketplace. It was *not*, in other words, only "the masses" who were interested in "other" medicine, nor was it just the lower classes who defended the rights of "other" healers. Lawyers and parliamentarians, police superintendents and regional governors, workers and artisans, publicists and political activists (and even some doctors) were active in their defense of the right of laypersons to practice medicine and in their belief that "unofficial" medicine should have a place among many competing medical models.[10] In the press and parliamentary debate, in association halls, rallies, and petitions, an extraordinary range of voices came together in defense of a free medical marketplace. While it is clear that professional interests were staked in the regulation of the medical marketplace, more abstract issues—the rule of law, the regulation of speech, and the development of science—were also in play.

This chapter charts various efforts to organize the medical marketplace in Germany after 1869, focusing in particular on the period after 1900. It is not intended as a comprehensive legal history, but rather as an attempt to understand how debates about regulation became intertwined with claims about individual rights and the freedom of scientific inquiry. The defense of the free medical marketplace transcended differences of class, profession, and political party. Because of natural healing's growing popularity, particularly in the period after 1890, the medical lobby encountered very strong head winds as it sought to regulate the practices of nonlicensed healers. By focusing not just on the defensive alliances that pitted medical associations against "other healers," but on the range of actors who made their voices heard, I hope to show that defenders of lay-healing traditions like *Naturheilkunde* came not just from the "gullible masses," as medical lobbyists argued.

Healing traditions like *Naturheilkunde* were legitimate players in a rich and varied medical marketplace. As we shall see in chapters 4 and 5, this had far-reaching consequences for the theory and the practice of medicine.

CHARLATANS AND SWINDLERS?

Calls for the increased regulation of the medical field appear to have stemmed, at least in part, from anxieties about the increased presence of nonlicensed practitioners in the urban landscape. An October 1897 report on the consequences of deregulation claimed that "the number of nonlicensed practitioners [*Pfuscher*] had never been so great."[11] In Berlin, for example, the report cited the presence of 476 nonlicensed practitioners, among them apothecaries, midwives, and orderlies.[12] If the increasingly frantic communications between local, state, and national officials are any indicator, the number of nonlicensed practitioners had, in fact, grown dramatically during the 1890s. A 1911 report claimed that, between 1879 and 1898, the number of nonlicensed healers active in Berlin had grown at a rate of 1,600 percent. Between 1901 and 1911, the numbers had grown a further 300 percent, rising from 2,404 to 7,549.[13] While these numbers are surely exaggerated,[14] they do point to the widespread belief that the practice of medicine by nonlicensed healers had expanded in troubling ways.

From the viewpoint of many local and regional administrators as well as police officials and civil servants during the *fin de siècle*, the free medical marketplace represented a public health risk. But regulations and initiatives to curb nonlicensed medical activity were fairly haphazard and lacking in uniformity from one region to the next. In Saxony, conviction for "quackery" carried with it a maximum penalty of 400 Marks or up to 40 days in jail,[15] while in Schleswig, the same crime warranted a fine of just 60 marks or a "corresponding jail term."[16] Administrators were acting in improvised ways because elected officials were unwilling to legislate the practices of nonlicensed healers: at various levels of government, elected officials believed that nonlicensed healers had as much right to practice as did university-trained doctors. As the *Kölnische Zeitung* told its readers in 1902, members of the Prussian Legislative Assembly were unwilling to restrict access to the free medical marketplace.[17] According to Minister of Ecclesiastical Affairs Konrad von Studt, the *Reichstag* was almost certain to reject increased regulation of lay healers.[18] Ultimately, as we shall see in the coming pages, medical lobbies were ineffective in their efforts to convince elected officials that nonlicensed healers were a danger to public health.

Given the lack of parliamentary support for a revision of the 1869 Trade Laws, officials at the Ministries of the Interior, Trade, and Ecclesiastical Affairs began developing a different strategy, one that would standardize the surveillance and punishment of nonlicensed healers.[19] The energy behind this new push for legislation came from the organized medical establishment, and a couple of market forces help to explain why this happened when it did. The well-documented overproduction of doctors was one important factor motivating medical associations in their efforts to curb competition.[20] Another less tangible factor was the changing media climate. While the medical marketplace had long seen growing competition between licensed medical doctors on the one hand and health and lifestyle entrepreneurs on the other, this pressure increased dramatically in the 1890s. One indication of this pressure is the spiking circulation rates of serial publications like *Nature's Doctor*, the explosion of popular health and hygiene publications, and the success of manuals like the ones published by Friedrich Eduard Bilz, Sebastian Kneipp, and others.[21]

While individual doctors did not typically turn to mass media outlets to shore up their market position, they did repurpose existing institutions, with some noticeable success. In 1898, for example, the journal *Gesundheitslehrer* was formed to educate the public about the dangers of "other healers." *Gesundheitslehrer* took the model of existing professional journals aimed at medical doctors and health care specialists and modified it to reach a broader audience. While the pieces appearing in the journal were typically authored by medical doctors, their tone and substance were more polemical than technical, making the journal accessible to laypersons and medical men alike.

Two years later, the *Schutzverband der Ärzte Deutschlands zur Wahrung ihrer Standesinteressen* was founded—as the name suggests—to protect the professional and economic interests of medical doctors. Widely known as the "Leipzig League," the *Schutzverband* joined with local medical associations (one historian uses the phrase "medical chambers of commerce") to influence insurance funds, legislators, and local administrators. These innovative strategies to protect the interests of licensed professionals were not, at first, universally popular. Historian Hedwig Herold-Schmidt has shown that older doctors in particular considered this kind of popular mobilization to be at odds with their "professional honor" or Standesehre.[22] These concerns were quieted by the Leipzig League's effectiveness in winning economic concessions from the insurance funds. Between 1900 and 1912, the League brought to a successful end 98 percent of the more than 1,000 negotiations in which they were involved.[23]

If the Leipzig League was very successful in winning support from medical professionals, it was far less effective in generating any broadbased popular support. Tactics like the "doctors' strike," modeled on the general strikes commonly associated with workers' movements, convinced many Germans that doctors were more concerned with their own professional interests than with the public good. The doctors' associations were hopeless at public relations, and in part because they failed to win popular backing for their initiatives, doctors and doctors' associations tended to appeal to the bureaucratic and administrative arms of the state rather than to the people or parliament.

This lack of public support for the medical profession was well recognized by contemporary observers. As a piece in Deutsche Warte explained, it was because doctors' demands for new rights and greater protections "found no echo with the people" that the profession sought help from state authorities. The author of the Deutsche Warte piece claimed that this appeal to state authorities could be explained by the fact that "doctors [were] represented in the state administrative apparatus in no small number."[24] Efforts to intensify regulatory controls on nonlicensed healers found limited support from elected officials, but they got a better reception in ministerial audiences.

On June 28, 1902, despite the political and legal challenges certain to face efforts to regulate the practices of nonlicensed healers, the Ministry of Ecclesiastical Affairs issued a series of decrees that would force nonlicensed healers to register with local medical officers. Recognizing that print media was an important vehicle for the spread of alternative therapies like *Naturheilkunde*, Konrad von Studt also tried to tighten the screws on the newspapers that carried advertisements for nonlicensed healers, giving medical officers and police officials the broadly defined power to fine newspapers for false advertising.[25] Nonlicensed healers would now face oversight from the very group that most wanted to limit their access to the medical marketplace.

Given their own professional interests, it is unsurprising that natural healing associations responded to these measures with alarm. The Associations of Practicing Natural Healers (*Vereine der Ausübenden Vertreter der Naturheilkunde*), for example, claimed that state regulation of the medical marketplace amounted to a "Chinese Wall" on the road to scientific progress, inhibiting the competition between different medical models and giving medical doctors what amounted to a professional monopoly. A different group wanted to know how the measures would be applied. What, they asked, would be the grounds for denying professionals permission to practice medicine?[26] Would medical doctors consider dangerous all treatment that deviated from accepted academy norms? As the VGN (*Verein für Gesundheitspflege und Naturheilkunde*) petition made clear, proposed measures gave medical doctors, "who already see the absence of a medical license as evidence of [the layperson's] unfitness for the healing trade," the tools to systematically persecute nonlicensed practitioners. In the face of widespread disagreement over scientific best practices, the VGN argued that health care decisions should be left to the patients themselves.[27] Copies of their petition were submitted to the Saxon Ministry of the Interior by 18 natural healing associations.[28]

Natural healing associations were not the only ones to raise concerns about Minister Studt's June 28 directives, and here we begin to see why medical lobbies had so much trouble marginalizing alternative practitioners. As the National Liberal newspaper *Kölnische Zeitung* noted, excluding swindlers and charlatans was a worthy goal, but introducing measures to police nonlicensed medical practices opened the door, in the eyes of many, to all manner of abuses. While ministry officials may have been justified in their anxiety about proliferating advertisements showcasing the abilities of "other healers" and their products, editorial writers for the *Kölnische Zeitung* thought that only uniform regulatory steps would ensure both press freedom (in choosing which advertisements to run) and the equal application of the law. The editorial staff took care to distinguish calls for caution from "an endorsement of quackery."[29] But how was the editorial staff supposed to judge the relative merits of one therapeutic regime over another—through laboratory testing of controlled substances and evaluations of individual healers? Or did the spirit of the police directives really demand that the medical qualifications of anyone advertising medical services be evaluated as part of the process of enforcing regulations? While the commercial interests of the press should not be ignored when evaluating its opposition to Studt's initiatives, the criticisms raised in the Cologne paper highlight the complicated legal questions facing advocates of increased regulation.[30]

Opposition from yet another quarter suggests that criticism of the June decrees was not simply an attempt by the press and natural healers to defend their economic interests. Just one day after the police directives were circulated to German dailies for publication, the Berlin Chief of Police, von Windheim, wrote a letter to Minister Studt arguing that there were no legal grounds for compelling nonlicensed healers to register with their local medical officers, and that directives covering the restrictions upon advertisement were completely outside the scope of police regulatory authority.[31] Von Windheim warned that similar attempts to effect policy through decrees had not withstood the scrutiny of higher administrative courts and that it was bad policy (and bad publicity) to put in place police directives that would later be overturned.[32]

This legal objection to the decrees was expressed from another angle and with equal force by the Hanover police chief Graf von Schwerin in a letter to the regional governor. Von Schwerin noted that paragraph 29 of the North German Trade Federation Act made clear its authors' intention to remove legal obstacles to the free practice of healing by any and all persons. In his view, the attempt to regulate advertisements, as well as the obligation to register one's trade with the local medical officer, was in direct conflict with both the spirit and the letter of the law. While the dangers of quackery were real, von Schwerin thought that unlawful rule by decree was ultimately more dangerous than allowing nonlicensed healers to practice their trade, which was a right ensured by the 1869 Trade Legislation.[33]

Reactions to the June decrees suggest that media elites and police officials were as concerned with the uniform administration of justice as they were with the specter of the swindler. Complaints about the "capriciousness" of the police directives and questions about the motives of medical doctors placed Minister Studt under considerable pressure, so much so that by December 1902 he felt compelled to revise the ministry's stance on advertisements. In a letter to regional governors dated December 31, 1902, Studt instructed police officials to warn editorial staff before issuing fines.[34]

Faced with widespread concerns over the implementation of police measures—concerns given voice not least by high-ranking police officials—ministry-level officials seem to have recognized that the only way to resolve the problem of "quackery" was to draft national legislation. Representatives of the Ministries of the Interior, Justice, and Ecclesiastical Affairs met on December 12, 1904, to discuss the proposed legislation, and the minutes of that meeting suggest that ministerial representatives were uncertain how best to implement more comprehensive regulation.[35] If the proposed law was not dead, it was moving forward less quickly than some would have hoped. The matter was still being debated in early 1908 when future Chancellor Bethmann-Hollweg weighed the merits of different strategies for managing the problem of nonlicensed healers.[36]

Opposition to the 1902 decrees demonstrates that efforts to regulate the medical marketplace failed to generate either enthusiasm or consensus, but as the following case shows, everyone involved in debates about the free medical marketplace recognized that some kind of reform was needed. In the following section, I use the famous "Felke Trial" to illustrate some of the challenges facing efforts to regulate the practices of nonlicensed healers. The Felke trial was a media circus that received widespread coverage throughout Germany. With its 27 expert witnesses and high-stakes debates, the trial was an amplified expression of similar proceedings that took place all over Germany.

PROSECUTING NONLICENSED HEALERS: THE FELKE TRIAL

On May 18, 1908, a 17-year-old baker's apprentice named Gerhard Ueltgesforth died of complications resulting from acute appendicitis. Eighteen months later, on Wednesday, October 27, 1909, the "biggest trial that the still young Crefeld district court had yet experienced" began, with Pastor Emmanuel Felke standing accused of negligent homicide.[37] According to testimony of his employer, Gerhard Ueltgesforth was already sick on Saturday morning, the 14th of May, and though he continued to work around the bakery, he went to bed early that evening, complaining of fatigue and abdominal discomfort. The following morning, despite being visibly unwell, Ueltgesforth set out on a weekend trip to visit his family, making the roughly three kilometers journey on foot. Over the next 24 hours, his condition worsened, and on Monday morning, his mother took him to the sanitarium of the renowned healer Pastor Emmanuel Felke. Felke was famous throughout Germany and typically saw between 30 and 40 patients each day. That morning, though, Ueltgesforth did not wait long, and after a brief examination—likely no more than a few minutes—Felke diagnosed Ueltgesforth with an inflammation of the liver,[38] prescribing a combination of homeopathic remedies, cool water baths, and his signature "Loam compress."[39] Ueltgesforth went home with his mother and followed Felke's directions.

By Wednesday morning, roughly 48 hours after his visit to Felke, the young man's condition had worsened dramatically. This time, his father telephoned the insurance-fund doctor in Homberg. It took most of the day to track down Dr. van Elsenberg, but when he was finally briefed on the patient's symptoms around 5 p.m., things moved very quickly. Ueltgesforth was transported the seven kilometers to the hospital, where he was rushed into surgery. He died later that evening from "a high-grade ulceration of the abdominal cavity."[40] Ueltgesforth's appendix had burst. This was the basic story, the details upon which both sides could agree. From these facts, the prosecution sought to prove that Felke had misdiagnosed Ueltgesforth, delaying surgical intervention. They further argued that this delay was responsible for the patient's death.

The defense did not dispute this timeline. Instead, they contested the prosecution's claim that surgery was indicated for the abdominal discomfort experienced by Ueltgesforth, or that surgery was the universally accepted treatment for appendicitis. They argued, in other words, that even if Felke had correctly identified Ueltgesforth's condition as appendicitis, the attending doctor would not necessarily have advocated surgical intervention. The defense used a combination of lay and expert testimony to make their case. On the one hand, they wanted to place Felke's track record front and center, forcing the judge to evaluate claims made by patients who were themselves convinced of Felke's extraordinary abilities. The defense also wanted to demonstrate that there were diverse strategies for treating appendicitis. In particular, they pointed to doctors who recommended a "conservative" approach to treatment. For the court to convict Felke, the prosecution would have to demonstrate that surgery *would* have saved Ueltgesforth's life. They would *also* have to prove—and this would be far more difficult—that any competent medical practitioner would have prescribed surgery.[41] The trial began with testimony about Felke's diagnostic methods.

According to Felke, one could identify illnesses ranging from liver disease to rheumatism simply through an examination of the irises. Felke learned of the "ocular diagnosis" (*Augendiagnose*) in the 1881 "Discoveries in the Field of Nature and Healing Arts" by the Hungarian doctor Ignaz von Péczely. Dr. Péczely claimed that the quadrants of the eyes—the right eye generally representing the right side of the body and the left eye the left side—corresponded to different regions and organs in the body. The top half of the iris, for example, corresponded to the brain, throat, heart, lungs, while the lower half indexed the liver, kidneys, intestines, genitals and so on.[42] The ocular diagnosis consisted of a careful observation of the patient's pupils and irises to identify anomalies in pigmentation. Based on their location, size, and coloration, these anomalies indicated pathologies in various parts of the body. In his testimony, Felke claimed that the "ocular diagnosis" was *sui generis*: "the diagnosis that I make from the iris has little to do with what one otherwise calls diagnosis. It accomplishes that which no other diagnostic can, without the patient ever having said a word."[43] When asked by the judge *how* he conducted the diagnosis, Felke said he simply looked into the patient's eyes, sometimes unassisted, sometimes with a magnifying glass. He told his audience that "one sees every change in the stomach, in the kidneys, in the bladder. It also explains [changes in] the different parts of the heart and lungs and so on. One can also see," he continued, "what medications have been used [by the patient]."[44] When asked by the judge whether he conducted any kind of physical examination, Felke replied that he did not. "Physical examination," he claimed, "would not give one tenth the certainty that the ocular diagnosis gives."[45]

In support of Felke's testimony, the defense produced a series of witnesses anxious to testify to his extraordinary competence. One of these was Herr Bellachini, a traveling magician from Marburg. Bellachini first visited Felke for chronic abdominal swelling. He had visited other doctors first, at least one of whom had prescribed a course of mercury therapy—a highly toxic "cure" once commonly prescribed for syphilis. His visit to Felke produced entirely different results. After a brief examination of his irises, the pastor explained that Bellachini was suffering from appendicitis. Warning him *against* surgery [!]—Felke told Bellachini that young doctors pushed surgery on unsuspecting patients because of the higher fees—Felke prescribed sitz baths, a vegetable and fish diet, and the loam compresses for which he was widely known. According to Bellachini, the prescribed cure worked wonders, with the inflammation rapidly subsiding. At the end of the verbal examination, Felke proceeded to show the assembled crowd the marks in Bellachini's eyes that indicated his appendicitis.[46] Medical experts for the defense testified that they could not be sure whether the pigmentation had any diagnostic merit. They did say that, given Felke's successful track record, his methods were worthy of systematic investigation.

The prosecution countered with expert testimony designed to discredit both the anecdotal evidence provided by lay witnesses like Bellachini and the testimony of expert witnesses for the defense. The eye specialist Dr. Seligmann, for example, provided exhaustive clinical research claiming that uneven pigmentation in the irises had no diagnostic significance.[47] Another witness for the prosecution, an eye specialist and contributing editor to *Gesundheitslehrer*, was equally critical. Dr. Neustätter had himself visited Felke's clinic in Repelen after he was criticized for rejecting the pastor's techniques without having taken the time to evaluate them first hand.[48] Accompanied by two medical colleagues, Neustätter visited Felke's clinic with the intention of submitting himself for a full evaluation. After a brief tour of the facilities, Neustätter invited Felke to conduct his eye exam, but not before warning him that he had recently taken several doses of a strong chemical compound as a clinical control to the experiment. Felke, after all, claimed that his diagnosis could identify not just sickness, but also the presence of harmful toxins in the bloodstream. Despite Neustätter's warning, Felke allegedly failed to identify any trace of the compound—a point that, in its own right, seemed to discount the veracity of his gaze. This was not, however, the only measure of his technique taken that day. Felke also examined one of Neustätter's companions and confidently diagnosed him with symptoms of "Bouillon-poisoning."[49] Neustätter's companion rejected the diagnosis, claiming that he had none of the symptoms, and when Felke tried to show Neustätter the clues that had pointed to his conclusions, the eye specialist claimed only to have seen "a very smooth . . . iris of dark grey coloring."[50] Neustätter told the court that "the ocular diagnosis is absolute humbug."[51]

Testimony by Seligmann and Neustätter, which was carefully reasoned, thorough, and often quite funny, seems to have been fairly effective in undermining confidence in the ocular diagnosis. It also shows just how far experts had to go to demonstrate the incompetence of "other healers." It is clear, for example, that both Neustätter and Seligmann thought the ocular diagnosis was nonsense, whether endorsed out of stupidity (as in the case of Bellachini), insanity (as in Felke's case), or the hope of financial or professional reward (as, presumably, in the case of the expert witnesses for the defense). The fact that Seligman and Neustätter nevertheless felt compelled to investigate the technique suggests that they understood how difficult it would be to convince the public of their point of view. As long as the defense was able to find medical doctors willing to testify to the possible merits of the ocular diagnosis, its critics would have to prove scientifically that the technique should be counted as "absolute humbug."

Having argued that there was no merit to the ocular diagnosis, the prosecution had still to prove that proper diagnosis would have resulted in life-saving surgical intervention. Here the question was whether or not early surgical intervention was indicated. Once again, expert testimony played an important role in the competing legal strategies. In support of their claim that early surgical intervention would have saved the patient's life, prosecutors cited medical experts who testified that patients receiving early surgical care had a survival rate upwards of 95 percent, a figure that decreased to 78 percent by the third day.[52] Expert witnesses for the defense rejected these findings. The medical doctor Dr. Rudolf Spohr, for example, testified that as long as the patient was able to move around under his or her own power, sitz baths could "frequently be applied to good effect."[53] According to his testimony, a conservative approach to treatment was preferable to early surgical intervention. Dr. med. Peter Ziegelroth, editor of the *Archive for Physical and Dietary Therapy*, claimed that Spohr succeeded 98 percent of the time using a conservative treatment. This point was used by the defense to refute the prosecution's claim that rapid surgical intervention provided the best outcomes in treating appendicitis. According to the defense, Spohr's success rate with noninvasive approaches was ample proof that "conservative treatment of the appendix is completely warranted."[54]

Attorneys for the defense telescoped in on cleavages within the medical community, raising doubts about the best course of medical action. To convict Felke, they argued, the judge would have to decide not just that surgery *would* have saved the patient's life if it had been prescribed. He would also have to decide that any competent medical practitioner would have recommended early surgical intervention if confronted with Ueltgesforth's case.[55] If even doctors disagreed over the proper course of treatment, how then could the court fault Felke for his decision? To find Felke guilty, the judge would have to adjudicate between competing medical models. Attorneys for the defense claimed that this was exactly what opposing counsel was trying to force him to do.

According to Dr. Schulze, attorney for the defense, the 1909 trial of Pastor Felke was not really about Ueltgesforth's death. Instead, prosecutors "had attempted to put the ocular diagnosis par excellence in the center of the trial."[56] Felke was being prosecuted "only because his views departed from those then current in medical science."[57] Questioning whether science was justified in characterizing Felke's methods of diagnosis as "humbug," Schulze invited the audience to look at "the annals of history," where science is on record as having often taken one side and defended its traditional views with "unbelievable stubbornness," "while on the other side are almost all the truly epoch-making discoveries," discoveries that the scientific establishment in many cases "foolishly" fought against for years.[58] By putting divisions within the medical field at the center of the trial, the defense successfully raised doubts about what constituted appropriate medical action in the Ueltgesforth case. According to the defense's argument, the prosecutors were attempting to penalize Felke for Gerhard Ueltgesforth's death and had created a case based upon prejudice and circumstance rather than on sound legal principles. As defense witness Dr. Emil Klein commented, "According to German law, [Felke] has right on his side." But, he sarcastically suggested, this hardly matters: "[S]imply make a new law!"[59] Klein was well known in natural healing circles, and in 1924 he was given a chair for physical and dietary therapies at the University of Jena. In this case, at least, he was wrong in his reading of the situation. The law did not change, nor was Felke convicted.

The only question that could convict Felke was whether he had *knowingly* proceeded in a negligent manner, and to this question, the judge replied in the negative. His statement is worth quoting at length: "In normal circumstances, the defendant can have had no doubt that the ocular diagnosis is an unreliable tool. Nevertheless, the court can not come to an affirmation of negligence, because the particular circumstances under which Felke practices his occupation in Repelen have to be taken into consideration. The whole milieu must be considered. . . . Perhaps in this milieu the defendant came to so certain a valuation of his healing method, that even the advice of doctors was not in a position to dissuade him from his firm belief."[60] The decision points to the extraordinary situation in which judges, police officials, and other regulatory officials were operating. In Germany's medical marketplace, negligence depended on knowledge. In a context of competing medical models, *knowledge was itself being contested*.

An opinion piece in the November 9, 1909, edition of *Der Tag* pointed to at least one problem facing regulators. If Felke was acquitted in large part because of his social position and his education, would it not be even more difficult to convict nonlicensed healers who did not have the kinds of advantages of education and upbringing that Felke had had? In these cases, proving ignorance would be even easier than it was in the Felke case. The Felke trial was a national event that demonstrated just how ineffective existing regulatory mechanisms were in organizing the medical marketplace. It highlighted the capriciousness of the system.

For critics of increased regulation, this case suggested that nonlicensed healers would continue to be persecuted because they did not have the "right" kind of credentials. Even though the court had, in this instance, decided in favor of the defendant, the decision created no precedent that would protect nonlicensed healers from similar trials in the future. The Felke case also bore out the worst fears of advocates of increased regulation of the medical marketplace. It suggested that, in the present regulatory environment, it would be impossible to effectively prosecute even those guilty of grievous crimes. The Felke trial stands as evidence of an impossibly incoherent system governing public health in Germany before the First World War.

LEGISLATING THE MEDICAL MARKETPLACE: PROGRESS AND PUBLIC HEALTH IN THE REICHSTAG

After much delay, draft legislation to regulate abuses in the healing trade was presented to the Royal Prussian Ministry of State on April 27, 1910. The proposed law had its first hearing in the 90th Session of the Reichstag on November 30, 1910, and the debate highlights many of the same issues we have seen so far. One of these was the tension between legislators and appointed state representatives. In his introduction to the proceedings, Undersecretary of the Interior Dr. Delbrück tried to reassure the assembled audience that proposed limits on the medical marketplace were designed to protect the public from negligence, not to prevent segments of the population from seeking help from unlicensed practitioners,[61] and not to create a professional monopoly for medical men. Although Delbrück's introduction attempted to enforce a narrowly framed debate centered on the rule of law, legislators from across the political spectrum were anxious to talk about a whole range of issues, from the nature of science and scientific progress, to civil liberties and freedom of choice. Delbrück's message was lost in a wave of competing viewpoints almost as soon as he finished his remarks.

Dr. Martin Fassbender, representative of the Catholic Center Party, was first to speak, and he made it clear that he was suspicious of the proposed legislation. Fassbender was well aware that many of his colleagues thought that the push for new regulatory controls was not about public safety, but about "the interests of doctors,"[62] and Fassbender agreed that there was some basis for that interpretation. Professional interest certainly played a role in calls for the increased regulations. Fassbender argued, though, that efforts to limit the free medical marketplace had deeper roots: doctors did not want to exclude lay healers just because doing so would enhance the power of medical associations. They also *believed* that university training should be a prerequisite for all healers and that progress in medicine would result from the concerted efforts of specialists and experts, not from the unsystematic work of laymen. The problem, of course, was that not everyone agreed with them. No small number of those skeptics happened to be sitting in parliamentary chambers.

It came as no surprise to anyone that advocates of natural healing and advocates of allopathic medicine disagreed about the pathogenesis of illness. What Fassbender also wanted to emphasize, though, was the fact that no clinical study or laboratory research had as yet demonstrated the superiority of one medical model over the other. For all the many advances in biology and chemistry—advances that had important consequences for anatomy, physiology, and pathology—doctors simply did not understand the human body well enough to justify their calls for a medical monopoly. In fact, medical doctors often had just as much trouble explaining their therapeutic successes as they did their failures. Fassbender argued that, as long as "university medicine" was in this early stage of development, it should continue to be tested in the marketplace of ideas. Participation in this marketplace of ideas should not be limited by one's educational, professional, or licensing background: the only limitations to participation should be a practitioner's ability to demonstrate the merits of ideas and practices in a competitive field.

Fassbender was aware that recent years had *also* seen a marked increase in the numbers of practicing charlatans. Was it possible, he asked, to target charlatans and quacks while ensuring protections for other healers?[63] Requiring nonlicensed healers to provide their business records to medical officers upon request, for example, seemed to Fassbender an extraordinary transgression of the individual right to privacy. (This point was received with calls of "quite right!" from the center.)[64] Perhaps a law to control the fraudulent practice of healing was necessary. More important, though, *"far more important than a law against quackery,* is doubtless the better education [*Aufklärung*] of the public about the condition of the body, about questions of nutrition, about cleanliness, the dangers of alcohol, and also education about the dangers of quackery."[65] In this regard and others, natural healing had made major contributions to medicine in its theory and practice.

It was clear almost from the outset that many legislators viewed the proposed law with suspicion. By the time the 32-year-old Social Democrat Fritz Zietsch took the floor, though, some themes were already becoming clear. Zietsch, like Fassbender, was concerned that the draft legislation threatened "not only to affect the true charlatans, but to reach far beyond."[66] In a point that drew widespread calls of "Quite right!" Zietsch asked, "But what is a *Kurpfuscher*? If one wants to combat *Kurpfuschertum* [quackery] on legal grounds, is it not then necessary to first define the term?"[67] In Zietsch's view, a *Kurpfuscher* was someone who practiced healing without being up to the job, a definition that, as he pointed out, had nothing to do with the question of licensing or education. "But one finds such people in all other trades, *without therefore having felt obliged to proceed against them legally."*[68]

In order to secure a virtual monopoly on the practice of medicine, all doctors and medical lobbies had to do was to convince the public "that anything learned on the basis of practical experience" rather than "through so-called academic training [*Schulweisheit*] . . . is to be designated as suspect."[69] In Zietsch's view, the defenders of licensed medicine were out to prove that anyone practicing medicine without a medical degree was a *"Kurpfuscher."* As the Social Democratic representative reminded the assembled audience, though, this definition was at odds with the spirit and the wording of the 1869 trade legislation. In what amounted to a slander of the thousands "that practice healing with the utmost honesty"[70]—a characterization met with calls of "Quite right!" from the Social Democrats—doctors were pushing a law based largely on professional self-interest. It was clear, at least to Zietsch and those who cheered him on in his remarks, that in "untold thousands of cases, Naturheilkunde has demonstrated its value."[71] The law, said Zietsch, "will not find the approval of the parliament, because ... Naturheilkunde might in this way be destroyed [totgeschlagen] with a single blow."[72] In Zietsch's view, the Reichstag was not the place to adjudicate the relative merits of Naturheilkunde and academic medicine.

There were, of course, supporters of the proposed legislation. Expressing surprise at attacks on the proposed law, the eye doctor and National Liberal from Hanover, Wilhelm Arning, departed from his planned comments to defend his profession from perceived attacks and to speak of the pressing need for legislative initiative on the part of his colleagues. While acknowledging that medicine was indeed an art, and that there were, in some rare cases, individuals gifted with a natural ability that had nothing to do with training or education, he also argued that the law was designed to deal with the general rule, and not its exception. In Arning's view, swindlers attempting to defraud the gullible of their hard-won wages were the norm rather than the exception.[73] In a telling anecdote, Arning claimed that a medical officer in his district had reported that as many as half of all nonlicensed healers under his surveillance had been convicted of infractions against the penal code. Another conversation had disclosed the fact that "notorious lunatics" were to be found among the ranks of the lay healers.[74] Raising the specter of unregulated swindlers and criminally insane confidence men populating the ranks of the nonlicensed healers, Arning claimed that strong legislation was required to control the situation. His colleagues were not convinced.

When hearings began again on the next day, Dr. Mayer of the Center Party reiterated many of the points made by representatives from other party factions. While Mayer agreed that an "adequately funded medical estate" was essential to the welfare of the nation,[75] he rejected the view, taken by some advocates of increased regulation, that this could only be achieved by the exclusion of nonlicensed healers from the medical marketplace. "The proscription of . . . the freedom to choose one's healer [Kurierfreiheit] means at the same time a proscription of civil freedom more generally. . . . Here it is a question of the right [to control] one's own body."[76] As a member of the Catholic Center Party, and with the memory of the Kulturkampf still just decades old, Mayer recognized how dangerous it was to have the state intervene in questions of personal conscience, in beliefs about life and the body. If rational citizens believed that one kind of therapy was more effective than another, or that a nonlicensed healer could more effectively provide therapy than his or her licensed counterpart, what, he asked, were the legal grounds to intervene in that relationship?[77] Social Democratic representative Stücklen, and National Liberal Dr. Stresemann echoed Mayer in claiming that the proposed legislation would limit the choices available to patients and constitute a gross intrusion in a sphere of personal freedom. One of the most interesting things about this parliamentary debate was the way it escaped the logic of party affiliation, with representatives speaking for and against the proposed legislation without regard to their party allegiances. As Wilhelm Lattmann of the German Social Party pointed out, ". . . no party took a principled position [about the legislation], either negative or positive."[78]

The weeks following the first parliamentary hearing saw widespread press coverage of the proposed legislation, and debates in the press bear striking similarities to the parliamentary debate. On December 1, the Deutsche Tageszeitung worried that the proposed law would indiscriminately affect all nonlicensed healers without improving public health.[79] The law failed to draw distinctions between "other healers" who rejected the principles of orthodox medicine and the quacks and charlatans who endangered public health. In their report one week later on a public meeting at the Germania Hall on Berlin's Chaussee Straße, the Berliner Tageblatt echoed concerns raised in the Deutsche Tageszeitung. Describing a crowd of some 2,000 people, and the flurry of 300 telegrams posted from all over Germany, the author claimed that the crowd was convinced that the present law would open "[both] [g]ate and door to hateful denunciations."[80] The very vocal crowd "[saw] in the draft law a thoroughly unsuitable measure for pulling the floor out from under the true quacks, because these [could] only be destroyed through . . . the education of the people."[81]

Opposition to the law came from a number of different quarters, but medical associations did little to counter the objections of the law's critics. In fact, the medical associations themselves attacked some of the law's provisions, particularly the "compulsion to provide care" (*Kurierzwang*), which made it obligatory for doctors to treat patients who were in need of immediate medical attention. Hostility to the so-called *Kurierzwang* had been an important part of medical association platforms for more than four decades and played a catalyzing role in the creation of the free medical marketplace in 1869. At that time, the Berlin Medical Association pushed the North German Free Trade Act, in part to free medical doctors from a whole range of professional responsibilities, chief among them, the "compulsion to provide care." But freedom came with a price. If doctors were unwilling to provide medical attention on demand, then patients must have the freedom to seek care from a willing provider. As an editorial in the *Nationale Zeitung* put it in 1900, if "the state fails to ensure [medical] care for all, it cannot deny the right to seek assistance" from nonlicensed persons.[82]

Parliamentary hearings echoed these points, now almost a decade old. As committee members Stadthagen, Stücklen, and Zietsch made clear in riders to the legislation, a return to the 1869 *status quo ante* was only possible if doctors submitted to the so-called "compulsion to provide care." Why was this stipulation such a sticking point for both sides? Because the so-called *Kurierzwang* acted as a potential check on a medical monopoly, a check ensuring that patients would receive adequate care even if doctors tried to use their control over the medical marketplace to extort wage concessions or other professional advantages. As we will see in the next section, this was not just an academic point. Doctors *had*, in fact, repeatedly withheld care in exactly this way. For some elected officials, the "compulsion to provide care" clause was a way to ensure that doctors' associations could not use their monopoly to manipulate the marketplace by choking off access to an essential service.

As one might expect, the measure introducing the *Kurierzwang* as a condition for revision of the 1869 law met with a storm of protest from medical associations, including letters from the Saxon State Medical Council, the Württemberg State Medical Association, the Medical Association [*Ärztekammer*] of Baden, the State Medical Association of Hessen, the State Medical Association of Mecklenburg, and the Assembly of Doctors and Apothecaries, Braunschweig.[83] The unwillingness of medical associations to accept this set of responsibilities as a condition of their medical monopoly put them at odds with some of the same ministry officials who were championing their cause. The ineffective public relations work done by medical associations like the Leipzig League goes some way toward explaining why efforts to control the medical marketplace had so little success.[84]

It is clear that proposed legislation faced a difficult road. There were also powerful actors who supported new and tighter regulation of non-licensed healers, though not necessarily for the same reasons advanced by medical men. One supporter was Chancellor Bethmann-Hollweg, who believed that the free medical marketplace was compromising the state in its ability to manage women's reproductive resources. In Bethmann-Hollweg's view, natural healers were (in part) responsible for Germany's declining birth rates. He was not alone in thinking that charlatans, swindlers, reformers, and various other questionable characters were teaching women how to prevent conception or to terminate unwanted pregnancies. For medical associations, the issue of reproductive rights was a perfect vehicle for their campaign to control the medical marketplace. As Cornelie Usborne has argued, "Abortion proved a suitable platform for academic medicine to discredit and marginalize lay healers."[85] The image of the unscrupulous healer became linked with more general anxieties about population politics.

POPULATION STASIS, DOCTORS' STRIKES, AND THE COLLAPSE OF REFORM LEGISLATION

Attempts to control women's reproductive resources appear to transcend time and space, appearing not just in so-called modern societies, but also in petty-capitalist Qing modes of production[86] and Ndembu rituals.[87] If these kinds of efforts appear in a range of different social formations, though, the way these efforts were organized varied according to place and time. Mary Lindemann, for example, has shown how the regulation of sexuality intensified across the eighteenth century, and the nineteenth century saw this process continue. With advances in the study of demography, hygiene, and population sciences, efforts to control women's sexuality and their reproductive resources became closely tied both to medico-scientific discourses about social questions and efforts to professionalize the medical marketplace. Controlling women's reproductive resources meant, among other things, controlling the practices of nonlicensed healers.

The relationship between medical professionalization, reproductive resources, and the practices of nonlicensed healers can be seen, for example, in 1903 and 1904, when the regional medical officer for Bautzen bei Dresden noted an increase in the reporting of miscarriages. While Doctor Streit was unable to determine the cause of this troubling new situation, he suspected that "it had something to do with the striking number of natural healers, masseurs, etc."[88] While Streit admitted that the evidence was anecdotal, he also thought it was a matter of real concern. Streit urged health officials to alert doctors and midwives to the potential connection between the practices of nonlicensed healers and the growing incidences of suspicious terminations of pregnancy. "In cases of miscarriage," doctors and midwives "could investigate whether the woman in question had found herself in the care of a natural healer, masseur, magnetopath or some such."[89] Streit also thought it was important to alert professional associations to the potential public health risk, a recommendation that points both to the close relations between local medical officers and professional associations, and to the difficulty this could cause for nonlicensed healers.[90]

The Saxon State Medical Council supplied the Ministry of the Interior with its own view of the matter on February 8, 1906, and the report shows how concerns about population growth, anxieties about emancipated women, and the desire to regulate nonlicensed healers intersected. The council claimed that nonlicensed practitioners were being solicited not only for contraceptive medicines that could cause lasting harm to a woman's reproductive system, but also for information that would empower women to themselves induce miscarriages. This was particularly the conclusion (so said the council) of midwives, who believed that "the significant increase in the number of miscarriages" was a result of premeditation on the part of some women, who had in several cases "artificially induced" miscarriage.[91] Older midwives in particular had expressed their astonishment over the interest shown by married and unmarried woman in their reproductive physiology. The midwives claimed that women were using "whatever means available to prevent a pregnancy, and when they had not succeeded in this, to induce a miscarriage."[92] The report also asserted that women were getting this information in part by canvassing their peers, "in part through books, and in part by listening to lectures in natural healing associations."[93] Cornelie Usborne has shown that, before the war, women were significantly more likely to self-induce miscarriages than they were after the war, when pregnant women increasingly sought abortions from caregivers.[94] Even if lay healers were not directly responsible for the high incidence of aborted pregnancies noted in the 1904 and 1906 reports, the medical council suggested that nonlicensed practitioners were nevertheless at the root of the problem. By giving women the tools and the information to act on their own, unscrupulous quacks were contributing to Germany's perceived demographic crisis.

Bethmann-Hollweg's concern with the issue of nonlicensed healers seems to have evolved along precisely this axis, and it is possible that he would even have seen a copy of the 1906 report when serving as Minister of the Interior. Whatever the cause may have been, when legislation to regulate the medical marketplace was introduced in 1910, it contained a clause, written at the chancellor's behest, designed to significantly reduce the trade in substances necessary to prevent or terminate a pregnancy.[95] The regulation of nonlicensed healing, in other words, had support at the highest level of the German government. Those in search of intensified regulatory controls had a perfect vehicle for pushing their agenda, and a supporter willing to circumvent the messy conflicts that defined the Reichstag's 12th legislative period.[96] Subsequent decisions taken by the Leipzig League (*Schutzverband*) suggest, however, that doctors failed to understand that they needed to maintain the support of powerful allies if they hoped to build a monopoly in the medical marketplace. Their relationship with Bethmann-Hollweg, a key advocate for increased regulation of the medical marketplace, became a casualty of the Leipzig League's efforts to secure immediate economic gains.

Insurance Funds, Doctors' Strikes, and Bethmann-Hollweg

Since at least 1904, the relationship between medical associations (led by the Leipzig League) on the one hand and regional insurance funds on the other had become increasingly tense, as medical associations fought for increased honoraria and greater flexibility in their relations with the funds. Because insurance funds were obliged to provide medical attention to their members, a well-organized strike put them in a legally precarious situation.[97] If insurance funds failed to supply a certain number of doctors within a specified time frame, government arbitrators would open direct contract negotiations with the medical associations, to the pecuniary advantage of the doctors.[98] The Leipzig League was astoundingly successful in staging these strikes. Not only was it able to prevent doctors from crossing "picket lines": it was also able to negotiate favorable terms for its members with considerable consistency. In the period 1900–1912, the Leipzig League had a near-perfect record in bringing conflicts with local and regional insurance funds to a successful end.[99] A well-known 1904 case illustrates how these kinds of conflicts unfolded.

In March of that year, Leipzig doctors went on strike in search of higher honoraria. At the time the strike began, the Leipzig insurance fund had 235 doctors contracted to provide care to their members. When doctors struck, the Leipzig insurance fund tried to bring in doctors unaffiliated with the Leipzig League. The fund made offers around the country, offers that included, among other things, moving costs, high wages, and extended contracts. In spite of these very attractive offers, the fund was unable to attract the 98 doctors it needed to meet a minimum threshold for the provision of care. Patients encountered reduced services, high wait times, and other inconveniences. By the middle of April, government arbitrators were threatening to step in, and in the end, they did.[100] Huerkamp describes the five-week-long Leipzig doctors' strike as a "complete victory" for insurance-fund doctors, with all of their wage demands being met.[101]

If the Leipzig League was impressive in its ability to wrestle financial concessions from insurance funds across Germany, it was less effective in public-relations work. While the Leipzig strike may have been a "complete victory" in the short term, for example, Huerkamp points out that doctors "had to accept the tarnishing of their public image."[102] Not only did the doctors' strike color public perceptions of doctors and poison the relationship between medical associations and the insurance funds, it also colored the way that elected officials evaluated proposed limits on the right to offer health care services.

During the 153rd session of the *Reichstag* in 1905, the Social Democrat and insurance-fund administrator Julius Fräßdorf brought up recent events in Leipzig, Dresden, and Cologne. When doctors went on strike on April 1, 1904, Fräßdorf told the assembled audience, "all help, even for the seriously ill, was refused. Women were left bleeding, and members of the insurance funds have told me that they got down on their knees" begging for help. Fräßdorf cited a letter from a doctor who reported that "a workman had come to him with a brass fragment in his eye. Doctors at the royal clinic refused him aid, because he was a member of the municipal insurance fund." For Fräßdorf, this example showed how far doctors would go in order to protect their pocketbooks. Nor, he claimed, did these kinds of things happen just in Leipzig. Fräßdorf cited an article from the *Vössische Zeitung*, a newspaper that was "sympathetic" to doctors, detailing similar stories that emerged from the Mülheimer doctor strike. In this case, it was not a worker with a brass fragment in the eye, but a young boy with a broken arm.[103]

These kinds of stories are difficult to verify one way or the other, but the aggressive polemic of doctors' associations suggests that such scenarios were likely. One doctor wrote in a Leipzig newspaper, "It is good that we are free from the insurance-fund patients. At least we are away from the filth and the fleas."[104] Herold-Schmidt points to a similar example from 1900, in which a contributor to the *Ärztliche Vereinsblatt* wrote, "Out with the tyranny of the proletariat!"[105] Ongoing confrontations between the Leipzig League and insurance funds around Germany, combined with the "extreme and polemical style" of a significant number of editorials at the time, helped to create a wellspring of negative feeling toward medical doctors that would ultimately affect their professional opportunities over the long term.[106] Doctors' strikes poisoned the relationship between the profession and the public. It was against this backdrop that elected officials would, in 1910, debate proposed changes to the 1869 Free Trade Act.

"Verärgerte Terroristen": Final Negotiations

In early 1909, despite the open secret that new legislation to regulate the medical marketplace was soon to have a fresh reading in the Reichstag, doctors in Cologne went on strike in pursuit of higher wages and greater flexibility in the appointment of medical staff. The strike created a storm of unfavorable publicity, with political figures, the press, and various interest groups expressing their outrage over this strategic blackmail. One incident, in particular, seems to capture the extraordinary situation that was developing. As the *Rheinische Zeitung* reported, "A construction worker in Cologne-Lindenthal, who was seriously injured in a fall, was forced to wait five hours in excruciating pain, before assistance arrived. Eight doctors refused their assistance, and an insurance-fund doctor could not immediately proceed to the scene."[107] Little wonder, then, that doctors' calls for a more regulated marketplace *and* freedom from *Kurierzwang* were received with such skepticism. While the German Medical Association supported Cologne doctors in their efforts to secure better wages, the public reaction was far from favorable. Doctors' strikes highlighted some of the dangers that came with a medical monopoly.

Doctors' strikes were an exceptional case, and while Bethmann-Hollweg was an advocate for greater controls on the medical marketplace, he nevertheless felt compelled to condemn the Leipzig League's tactics. Not only did strikes endanger public health and safety, but they also put undue pressure on the relationship between doctors and the insurance funds, a relationship that was central to the provision of health care to millions of insured Germans. The *Berliner Tageblatt* reported that Bethmann-Hollweg was so concerned that he had even considered state intervention to compel doctors back to work, using strike-breaking regulations typically reserved for socialist labor associations.[108]

One Cologne medical association responded in no uncertain terms. In a strongly worded statement bound to lead to escalation, the association's members expressed their doubts about Bethmann-Hollweg's mental competence. Now they had gone too far, and parties not even directly involved felt compelled to comment. In an article titled "*Verärgerte Terroristen*," the *Leipziger Volkszeitung* reported on the ongoing saga, suggesting that "[e]nraged that this time, the state authorities did not unconditionally support their selfish endeavors as they had done in earlier years, the Gentlemen [the striking doctors] have laid their cards on the table."[109] Given the high-profile role the Leipzig League played in the strikes, it makes sense that Bethmann-Hollweg addressed his response to them. In a remarkably restrained letter to the Leipzig association, he claimed that when medical associations tried to blackmail their colleagues to strike, and when they tried "to make medical care conditional on the fulfillment of particular economic demands," they created dangers not only for the public, but for the medical estate as well.[110] The Leipzig association was reported as replying, "The German medical establishment is . . . armed for a battle to the death [*Kampf bis aufs Messer*], if real efforts are made to act on its economic organization."[111] While it is unclear how exactly this out-and-out conflict shaped the hearing of proposed legislation, it would certainly have made more difficult an already chilly political climate, raising doubts about the public-mindedness of associations pushing for passage of the law, and highlighting some of the dangers of a medical monopoly.

A strength of the proposed law was that it addressed regulators' anxiety about unlicensed and unregulated healers, fears of a population crisis, and suspicions that charlatans and confidence men were using the absence of regulation to defraud the German public. But doctors had done little to leverage this support for the purposes of ensuring the law's passage. Instead they antagonized important officials, the popular press, and public opinion with their aggressive defense of largely material interests. In the end, though, it was doctors' unwillingness to compromise on the issue of "compulsion to provide care" that led to the bill's failure. When revised legislation came out of committee in 1911, the Saxon State Medical Council declared itself decisively opposed to the amendment that reintroduced a limited "compulsion to provide care." Their reasoning was that the amendment *would impact negatively upon trust between doctors and patients!*[112] So soon after the horror stories coming out of the strikes, this justification would have had limited currency. While Bethmann-Hollweg continued to support tighter controls on the practices of nonlicensed healers and on the sale of abortifaciants, it is unlikely that he had forgotten the public insults thrown at him by the Committee Advocating Patients' Right to Choose a Doctor or the threatening language used by the Leipzig League.

In its New Year's edition for 1912, the editorial staff of *Nature's Doctor* noted with satisfaction that the law to introduce new restrictions on the medical marketplace remained, for now, "buried in . . . commission."[113] This was an important victory for natural healing associations and their roughly 150,000 members, and the arguments made by defenders of the free medical marketplace—in favor of freedom of choice, a marketplace of ideas, and the rule of law—clearly had something to do with the failure of the law to reach a floor vote in parliament. Perhaps equally important, though, was the failure of medical associations to recognize and exploit important tactical allies, or to effectively refute arguments made by their opponents. It may be that the doctors so badly underestimated the importance of public opinion and legislative goodwill because of their own high opinions of themselves and the work they did. Their apparent arrogance was also certainly bound up with their faith in (institutional) science and their belief that natural healing and other kinds of lay healing would eventually disappear, to be replaced by modern scientific practices. Whatever their thinking may have been, it is clear that the defeat of the November 1910 legislation taught them a lesson about the importance of good publicity in the age of mass publics.

CONCLUSION: THE WAR

The 1911 defeat of the law is not, of course, the end of the story. While there continued to be some space for maneuvering until at least May 1935, when all healers were subordinated to the 3rd Reich's Working Group for the New German Medicine [*Neue Deutsche Heilkunde*], things had already started to change in 1915. In the fall of that year, wartime censorship laws were used to prevent delivery of *Nature's Doctor* to field hospitals, lest patients be encouraged to demand natural therapies in place of the standard practices in military hospitals. One member of the

German League for Natural Healing later reported that "the word 'nature' acted on professional doctors like a red-flag," while another lamented the "difficulties confronting many colleagues in the simple attempt to apply moist compresses."[114] On the prerogative of some military governors general, and at the urging of the Ministry of War, natural healers were forbidden to treat sexually transmissible and infectious diseases in combat zones,[115] lectures were proscribed, pamphlets and fliers concerning the prevention of illness in the field were confiscated, and agitation against compulsory vaccination carried the danger of official sanction.[116] The war, then, accomplished at least partially what decades of agitation by doctors' associations had failed in peacetime to do. As with so many other segments of the home front, where civil liberties fall victim to the exigencies of war, debates about science and progress, the rule of law, and the right to free speech were swept away within a month.

If the First World War introduced constraints to the medical marketplace that decades of medical association lobbying had been unable to achieve, this was not a reflection of public opinion. As we shall see in the next chapter, *Naturheilkunde* continued to enjoy not just widespread popular support, but also powerful institutional advocates. One thing, at least, is clear: doctors' associations failed in their efforts to convince legislators that nonlicensed healers should be treated as uneducated quacks who endangered public health. Natural healing and the so-called *naturgemäße Lebensweise* were too deeply embedded in Wilhelmine everyday life for this strategy to be effective. But although medical associations failed in their efforts to discredit "the competition" in the eyes of their contemporaries, they enjoyed more success in shaping the historical view of alternative healing.

Historians too often assume that nonconventional healers were increasingly marginalized because of advances in biomedical science: in other words, scholars posit an archaic medical system that was superseded by a more modern therapeutic regime. As we shall see in the coming chapters, such assumptions are incorrect. In fact, *Naturheilkunde* become a victim of its own success: the professionalization of alternative healing actually led to the marginalization of its practitioners.

CHAPTER FOUR

SCIENCE FROM THE MARGINS?
Naturheilkunde from Outsider Medicine
to the University of Berlin, 1889–1920

As we saw in chapter 3, the relationship between academic medicine and the natural healing movement deteriorated rapidly in the period between 1890 and 1914, with questions of professional authority, personal choice, and public safety all contributing to friction between the two camps.[1] Professional competition over scarce resources was one important reason: as medical schools turned out more trained doctors, and as ever greater numbers of laymen joined the medical marketplace, the job of securing one's livelihood was becoming increasingly difficult for medical men. It was understandable for licensed doctors to want to exclude lay healers from the medical marketplace, but why should trained doctors continue to reject the natural therapies that had proven so effective in practice?[2] Writing in the inaugural issue of *Nature's Doctor*, the schoolteacher-turned-natural healer Hermann Canitz offered an explanation.[3]

Canitz claimed that university-trained doctors were hostile to lay healers not just because they hoped to monopolize the medical marketplace.[4] Doctors actually *believed* that lay healers were quacks and charlatans. During their years in training, doctors were taught to believe that progress in medicine resulted not from the unsystematic work of laymen, but from the concerted efforts of specialists and experts. These young men were initiates into a profession whose disciplinary structures "made it nearly impossible to view natural healing with an objective, unclouded eye."[5] For young medical men, it became "second nature" to treat internal illnesses with medications and to think about disease more in terms of the symptoms than the sick patient: this, according to Canitz, is what they had been trained to do.[6] As medical students internalized the norms of their profession, as they bent to the pressure of established hierarchies, these students submitted to the authority of medical textbooks and inherited dogma and turned away from what they saw with their own eyes: nonlicensed healers delivering effective care on the open market.[7] Tensions between medical men and lay healers were, in the view of Canitz and others, more cultural artifact than evidence of base economic motivations.

But the fact that doctors were not acting purely out of self-interest did little to improve the lives of lay healers who were under attack from medical associations. When, for example, the medical man Dr. Wolff testified against Canitz in a trial for medical malpractice, he argued that because natural healers like Canitz rejected many of the findings of the latest medical science, an acquittal of the natural healer amounted to an indictment of medical science. He warned the court that if Canitz went unpunished, universities "might as well simply close the lecture halls."[8] In 1889, when Canitz wrote, medical men assumed that the very fact of being a natural healer meant that one rejected scientifically tested theories, that one challenged established social hierarchies, and that one practiced therapies that were at best useless, and at worst dangerous.[9] Even 20 years later, the contours of the debate appeared unchanged. Doctors' associations continued to trade insults with natural healing associations, and the professional stakes had, if anything, grown. If one looks more closely, though, the transformation of the situation was dramatic.

This chapter charts the changing status of *Naturheilkunde* from 1889 to 1920. When Canitz wrote his piece in 1889, medical lobbies and doctors' associations were still pushing the view that all natural healers were quacks and all natural healing quackery. They conflated the practices with the practitioners. By 1920 it had become increasingly common for university-trained doctors to use natural therapies in their daily practices. A change in attitude in the medical establishment had clearly taken place, but it does not follow that the medical lobby had changed its attitude toward lay healers, who were the primary practitioners of *Naturheilkunde*. In the view of the medical associations, the lay healers themselves were all quacks.

This chapter is about another of those ways that *Naturheilkunde* remained a vital part of the German medical landscape. In chapter 2, we saw the role new consumer cultures and publicity networks played in popularizing natural therapies. Chapter 3 explored the unexpected alliances that formed to defend the free medical marketplace, highlighting the range of political, legal, and scientific arguments that were at play when debating who would be allowed to practice medicine. In this chapter, I explore a different dimension of the strange story that saw a Social Democratic minister of culture calling for the creation of professorships for natural therapies at German universities. This chapter might be seen as a story not just of survival, but of the triumph of *Naturheilkunde*.

If this chapter charts *Naturheilkunde*'s entry into the university establishment, it also tries to highlight what was lost in that process. While the creation of chairs for natural therapies at German universities elevated the status of *Naturheilkunde* as a set of practices, creating a *de jure* parity with other healing traditions like allopathic medicine, it did nothing to change the attitudes of medical lobbies and doctors' associations to their nonlicensed colleagues. Natural therapies were integrated into the academy while doctors' associations continued to demonize nonlicensed practitioners as quacks and swindlers. Paradoxically, the success of natural healing associations in pushing for better and more standardized training ended up reinforcing the attitude that university training should be a necessary condition for practicing medicine. Credentials began to matter more than practitioners' abilities.[10] This shift in attitudes had real consequences. As we saw in chapter 1, one core premise of *Naturheilkunde* was that anyone with a reasoned mind who was willing to observe the natural world carefully could be a healer. The lay quality of the natural healing movement was, in some ways, central to the kinds of therapies that natural healers advocated.

Professionalizing the practice of natural healing had another consequence. In the course of the nineteenth century, natural healers and lifestyle entrepreneurs made the case that health was not the result of medical silver bullets that treated individual symptoms, but rather the sum total of thousands of daily practices. This is why natural healers and other Life-reformers were concerned with everything from diet and exercise to sexuality and education, from clothing and leisure to political issues—like the ventilation of work spaces and access to adequate housing and urban green space. *Naturheilkunde* was essentially holistic in its outlook, and this holistic quality is one of the things that distinguished it from other healing traditions. As *Naturheilkunde* was integrated into the medical establishment, the holistic principles that made it unique began to disappear. Paradoxically, it was the popular pressures to establish university chairs for natural therapies that contributed to this process.[11]

"THERAPEUTIC NIHILISM" AND THE "CRISIS OF MEDICINE": MEDICAL MEN TURN TO "OTHER HEALING"

Viewed from a macrohistorical perspective, the trajectory of medicine in the last 150 years looks a bit like a steadily ascending arc—with the discovery of the tuberculin bacillus and the introduction of morphine, penicillin, and advances in imaging technology all plotted as important points or markers along the way.[12] This perspective has been critical in shaping the way that those of us looking back have come to think about allopathic medicine—alternatively called conventional, clinical, or Western medicine—and about lay alternatives. What gets erased in this kind of story is the limited impact that "medical innovation" actually had on the routine interactions of patients and doctors.[13]

Certainly until the widespread introduction of penicillin during the Second World War, therapy and treatment lagged far behind classification and diagnosis, and this gap helps to explain why patient confidence in their doctors was so low.[14] When confronted with the "big killers" of the nineteenth century, including smallpox, tuberculosis, and cholera, the situation was particularly grim. In the face of these kinds of diseases, doctors were still almost powerless, a fact that was recognized by the millions who "experienced this helplessness on their own bodies."[15] It was ultimately this tension between doctors' claims to professional authority and their inability to intervene on the patient's body

that was responsible for a "crisis of medicine."[16] If contemporary reports
are to be believed, the public was well aware that doctors promised far
more than they could deliver.[17] While doctors were increasingly able to
identify disease and to chart its likely course, they could still do little
to cure their patients. Young doctors in particular lamented the "therapeutic nihilism"[18] that characterized their discipline. In the late nineteenth century, a desire to provide better medical care at the bedside
led some young doctors to explore alternative therapeutic regimes.[19]
Some newly minted doctors began to consider alternative healing
traditions as a possible antidote to therapeutic nihilism. Because of
its extraordinary popularity, *Naturheilkunde* offered a particularly attractive professional outlet for doctors anxious to tap into an expanding sector of the medical marketplace.

We know that until at least the 1840s, doctors from across Europe
had visited Prießnitz in Gräfenberg to study his methods, but in the
period after 1850, this exchange of ideas across professional boundaries began to dry up. By the 1890s, medical men had long neglected the
work of their nonlicensed colleagues in the natural healing movement,
staking their hopes instead on a more mechanistic view of the human
body.[20] In a number of ways, this decision had paid dividends. Technical
innovation and increasingly precise diagnostic methods made German
medicine the envy of the world. Still, if the bet had paid dividends, it
also had costs. The intensifying focus on laboratory research had some
doctors wondering what had happened to their vocation as healers, and
they began calling for greater attention to patient care.

In this context, medical journals emerged that gave voice to the belief
that physical and dietary therapies could provide a useful corrective to
a medical science too long confined to the laboratory. For a variety of
reasons, this shift was extraordinarily important for the natural healing movement. Among other things, having doctors who championed
natural therapies made it more difficult for medical associations to
claim that only the uneducated masses preferred *Naturheilkunde* to
"university medicine." The challenge for medical associations trying to
marginalize natural healers became more difficult with the founding of
two medical journals dedicated to the scientific study and application
of natural therapies.

The *Archive for Physical and Dietary Therapy* (*ApdT*) was founded in 1899 by Dr. Peter Ziegelroth, who hoped to create a forum for testing the effectiveness of natural therapies and to educate the public about nonchemical alternatives. Directed to twin audiences—medical men concerned with questions of therapeutic competence and a general readership anxious to take control of its own health—Ziegelroth linked the creation of *ApdT* to failures within the ranks of the medical establishment. He founded the journal, he claimed, because the doctors had exchanged medical prophylaxis and comprehensive treatment for "therapeutic skepticism and nihilism."[21] Advances in natural science and medical pathology were, in part, responsible for this situation. Ziegelroth argued that the tendency toward localization of illnesses and the reliance on chemical treatments gave rise to the mistaken belief that acting on symptoms amounted to the same thing as healing the patient. He certainly was not alone in raising these concerns. Some bacteriologists argued that an exclusive reliance on medicating patients was dangerous, and they advocated a multicausal approach that emphasized the importance of environmental factors and individual disposition in accounting for sickness and health. In this context, Ziegelroth and his colleagues viewed it as their mission to "battle the tyrannical rule of the prescription" by providing comprehensive articles about the "physical and dietary therapies" long associated with natural healing.[22]

Ziegelroth's archive, as it was sometimes called, was not the first scholarly journal to stress the importance of physical and dietary therapies. In 1898, the pathologist Ernst von Leyden and professor of medicine Alfred Goldscheider started publishing the *Journal for Dietary and Physical Therapy* (*ZdpT*). Though contributions to their journal came almost exclusively from academic and medical men, their injunction to doctors—treat the sick person and not the sickness—was a philosophy commonly associated with the natural healing movement.[23] Pointing to what they called the long-standing eclipse of therapy under the "sign of diagnostics," they expressed a desire to raise physical and dietary therapies to parity with other branches of academic medicine.[24] Here, once again, the excesses of academic medicine, and its strong bias toward the laboratory at the expense of therapeutic innovation, drove the search for medical alternatives into uncharted territory. The founding of *ApdT*

and *ZdpT* is one indication of the growing acceptance of natural therapies in the academic mainstream.[25]

The last years of the nineteenth century seem, at first, to mark an
important shift in the fortunes of the natural healing movement. As
growing numbers of doctors began to use therapies long advocated in
the pages of *Nature's Doctor*, the boundaries between the two medical
traditions became less rigid. While the *ZdpT* remained intentionally
aloof from lay healing circles, Ziegelroth's public acknowledgment of
the role played by laymen in the development of "physical and dietary
therapies" seemed to hold out hope of an important new alliance, one
that would lend cultural and institutional authority to the natural healing movement.

This assumption proved, at least in the near term, to be unfounded. In
summer 1900 the Board for Medical Ethics voted to fine doctors 2,000
Marks for lecturing to natural healing associations,[26] a move designed
to deter their members from collaborating with the lay healing movement. The situation deteriorated when in October, the Doctors' Association for Physical and Dietary Therapy (*AVpdT*) decided to refuse
contact with natural healing associations, and it appealed to all doctors, regardless of their sympathies for medical alternatives, to do the
same.[27] It seemed that the growing popularity of natural therapies, and
their heightened profile in medical circles, was not translating into an
endorsement of the lay healers who had done so much to develop and
popularize those therapies.[28]

If leaders of the lay healing movement were upset by the summer
decision of the Board for Medical Ethics, they were furious at this dis-
avowal by an organization that had seemed, at first, to be a potential
ally. In response to the *AVpdT* decision, the German League called on
members to boycott doctors who held membership in any organization that attacked the interests of the natural healing movement. The
Doctors' Association for Physical and Dietary Therapy (*AVpdT*) soon
reversed its position, removing restrictions on its members. In an effort
to improve relations with the German League, which after all provided
potential professional outlets for *AVpdT* members, the association's executive committee even went so far as to publicly declare its support for
the natural healing movement in its 1905 annual meeting in Frankfurt.

STRATEGIES TO MANAGE NONLICENSED HEALERS: CO-OPT THE PRACTICES, EXCLUDE THE PRACTITIONERS

As natural healing found allies among medical men, medical associations could no longer easily argue that natural therapies were based on ignorance and superstition. The medical lobby was forced to develop new ways of marginalizing natural healers. One strategy was to rewrite history so as to co-opt the contributions that had been made by natural healers. Beginning in the late 1890s, some within the medical establishment argued that natural therapies had long been part of their therapeutic arsenal, pointing to key figures in the medical canon—Hippocrates and Galen, for example—who had used water, sunlight, diet, and movement in their therapies. By pointing to forefathers of modern medicine who had used natural therapies, these revisionists hoped to show that "natural healing" was not a distinct medical ideology, but rather a subspecialty in the broader medical landscape. The revisionists hoped to make "alternatives" to the medical mainstream redundant.

At least one doctor thought that the time had come to highlight the common ground shared by *Naturheilkunde* and "university medicine" rather than to emphasize their differences.[29] In "A Proposal for Peace," published in *ApdT,* the author aligned himself with reform currents within the medical establishment, citing the frustration many doctors felt with the slow pace of therapeutic innovation. Like his colleagues at *AVpdT,* "Dr. W." tied his frustration to the strong bias toward laboratory research that, after roughly 1850, had come to dominate the medical establishment.[30] Pointing to changing attitudes among even the most vocal critics of natural therapies, though, he argued that medicine was being transformed: In the 1880s and 1890s, it had been common for medical associations to accuse natural healers of quackery and criminality. By 1905, when the Proposal's author was writing, medical men and medical associations were publicly acknowledging the usefulness of physical and dietary therapies. As more and more doctors began to see illness as a dynamic process, they also began to treat the patient in more holistic ways, focusing less on the symptom and more on the person.[31]

This change in attitudes did not mean that doctors were likely to adopt wholesale the therapies natural healers were advocating.[32] As

Dr. W. pointed out, when faced with traumatic injuries or terminal ill-nesses, doctors were not always in a position to prescribe noninvasive, holistic therapies, even if this is what they would like, ideally, to do. But these were the extreme cases, and Dr. W. was confident that his licensed colleagues would increasingly use nonchemical, noninvasive therapies wherever possible. After years of destructive conflict, the anonymous doctor argued, it was time to put aside partisanship on both sides of the debate. "*Naturheilkunde* and academic medicine have long since stopped being anathema to one another," he noted, and natural therapies provided an important tool for doctors anxious to enhance their therapeutic ef-fectiveness.[33] Once medical men and lay healers recognized this new situation, they could begin to move forward together. Natural healing was, in this view, an important subset of medicine more generally and a useful complement to existing therapeutic techniques.[34]

Dr. Franz Kleinschrod wrote a cautious response in the pages of *Na-ture's Doctor*.[35] As a licensed medical doctor with strong commitments to *Naturheilkunde* and to the traditional prerogatives of lay healers, Klein-schrod welcomed the possibility of easing tensions between the two tra-ditions. The prospect of increased funding for research and training was certain, in his view, to contribute to the improved standing of *Naturhe-ilkunde* in the medical landscape. But Kleinschrod argued that reconcili-ation would not be possible if reformers in the two camps tried to ignore fundamental differences between the two traditions. In this regard, the peace proposal was not a promising start. According to Kleinschrod, it showed that Dr. W. did not understand the basic principles of the natural healing movement. Dr. W. thought that *Naturheilkunde* was a set of prac-tices that could be used to complement medication, vaccination, sera, or surgery in order to improve therapeutic outcomes. Dr. W. was advocating an eclectic approach to therapy, and this is the version of *Naturheilkunde* that is widely practiced even today.

For Kleinschrod, Dr. W.'s proposal demonstrated his ignorance of *Naturheilkunde's* basic tenets. "Sickness," wrote Kleinschrod, "is not a mechanistic-causal process" in the way that allopathic doctors as-sume, "but rather a biological process that has as its goal the body's accommodation to the presence of harmful substances."[36] Dr. W.'s eclecticism ignored the holistic foundations of *Naturheilkunde*. And in

Kleinschrod's view, it was this holistic quality that distinguished natural healers from their allopathic colleagues. Kleinschrod argued that
differences between *Naturheilkunde* and mainstream medicine existed
not at the level of medication—with water, diet, and massage therapies prescribed instead of medication and the like—but at a systemic
level. In his effort to hybridize the two traditions, Dr. W. ignored the
holistic foundations of natural healing. Like many of his colleagues
in the natural healing movement, Kleinschrod believed that accept-
ing "peace proposals" seeking to downplay the fundamental differences
between the two healing traditions would, over the long term, reduce
natural healing to a subset of an allopathic medicine to which it was,
in essential ways, opposed. In this view, the rapprochement between
Naturheilkunde and allopathic medicine signaled the end of natural
healing as a distinct medical cosmology.

The "peace proposal" raised a serious dilemma for the natural healing movement. On the one hand, it promised to enhance the institutional legitimacy of physical and dietary therapies that doctors' associations and university professors had long tried to marginalize. In
part for this reason, though, the possibility of a reformed medicine
created new problems for the natural healing movement, threatening
to replace the holistic principle with eclecticism. Nor was the danger
of being co-opted the only one facing the natural healing movement
in the age of medical reform movements. Another approach bluntly
called for the exclusion of lay healers from the medical marketplace
as the condition for integrating natural therapies into the medical establishment.

Dr. Franz Bachmann, director of the Society for Biological Medicine, a group dedicated to reforming social hygiene and sympathetic to
physical and dietary therapies, agreed with calls for greater cooperation
between the natural healing movement and hygiene reform societies
like his own.[37] He echoed points made in the "peace proposal," claiming
not only that medical men had moved away from the "mechanistic therapies" of which natural healers were so critical, but also that they were
starting to embrace the physical and dietary therapies that the natural
healing movement had long advocated.[38] In light of this transformation
of the medical field, Bachmann claimed that members of his society

were open to all natural therapeutic techniques and innovations. The Society for Biological Medicine was ready "to adopt [these innovations] without regard for dominant tendencies and authorities [in medicine]" if, for their part, lay healers would leave the practice of physical and dietary therapies to the experts.[39] The natural healing movement and the Society for Biological Medicine could, according to Bachmann, join forces as soon as the former agreed to dispense with "the ruinous practices of self-healing [selbstkurieren] and quackery [queckselber]"[40] that had, in his view, long characterized lay healing. He and his colleagues were excited about Naturheilkunde as a set of practices. However, they were not prepared to work with lay healers.

On the surface, Bachmann's "Way to Peace" [Weg zum Frieden] and the anonymously published "peace proposal" look roughly the same, and they do overlap in important ways. But while W.'s "peace proposal" worked to integrate natural therapies into an already existing arsenal of conventional treatments, making healers junior colleagues in an "eclectic" medical marketplace, it aimed to appropriate the practices of natural therapies while jettisoning the system behind it—its holistic principles. Bachmann's proposal, on the other hand, promised to view Naturheilkunde as a system, so long as its lay practitioners could be forced to give up their "ruinous practices." In either case, alliances that seemed at first to benefit the natural healing movement threatened to transform Naturheilkunde in fundamental ways.[41]

Reinhold Gerling had recognized the dangers of this dual challenge almost a decade earlier—before AVpdT had made its show of solidarity, individual doctors had issued their peace proposals, or hygiene reform societies had promised future collaboration. The occasion for his criticism was Oswald Vierordt's 1897 call for the creation of a hydrotherapeutic clinic at the University of Heidelberg, where he was a professor of medicine. Vierordt's proposal was part of a broader trend, anticipating not only the founding of ApdT and ZdpT, but also the creation of an autonomous section for Balneology at the German Congress of Natural Scientists and Doctors in 1898. Even so, it represented an early departure from an establishment consensus that sought to confine natural therapies to the fringes of the medical marketplace. As such, it was greeted with enthusiasm by the rank and file of the natural healing movement.

Gerling took a more cynical view. Why, he asked his readers, were they so anxious for this stamp of approval from the medical mainstream? Theirs was, after all, a hugely popular people's movement that had long championed the belief that knowledge was not the "privilege of a [medical] caste," but the right and responsibility of all citizens.[42] As they looked for validation for natural therapies in decisions taken by medical elites, important figures within the natural healing movement demonstrated how thin was their commitment to underlying principles of Naturheilkunde, which rested upon the assumption that the outlines of the universe were accessible through careful observation, through rational experimentation, and through experience. "What," he asked, "should [they] recognize? Our existence? That is not necessary. We exist! Our teachings? And who should recognize them? Science, for example? Which science? Do we not ourselves have access to the same scientific knowledge, to the same immutable truths that have been demonstrated through countless [therapeutic] triumphs? Is science not simply the apprehension of truth?"[43] Gerling reproached his fellows in the natural healing community for reacting positively to Vierordt's editorial: in his view Vierordt's proposal would ultimately produce hierarchies not only of knowledge, but of knowers. The natural healing movement adhered to the essentially populist belief in the rational individual's ability to know his or her own body. Ideas like Vierordt's were changing the movement from within and would present it with some real challenges.

In the first years of the twentieth century, the natural healing movement was guided by two, often competing, drives. The executive committee of the German League for Natural Living and Healing wanted to improve the training available to natural healers, create research facilities to speed the pace of therapeutic innovation, and build centralized outlets where patients could find treatment from healers trained in the practices and principles of Naturheilkunde.[44] But some of those voices demanding state support for research, training, and treatment were uncertain how much authority they were willing to cede to licensed doctors in an increasingly professionalized medical marketplace. The medical community's embrace of natural healing was changing Naturheilkunde in important ways, and the movement began to forsake some of its holistic principles in favor of an eclectic approach to therapy. Hierarchies began to emerge within a movement that had long been dominated by laypeople. In the first years of the twentieth century, natural healers, their patients, and advocates were forced to chart a course dictated by competing pressures. In a landscape marked by rapidly changing boundaries, where medical men embraced the practice of physical and dietary therapies while rejecting the lay practitioners who had pioneered them, it looked as though the broad dissemination of *Naturheilkunde* might only be achieved by the professionalization of its practices.

ALTERNATIVE MEDICINE AT THE ACADEMY. A CHAIR FOR *NATUR-HEILKUNDE* AT FRIEDRICH WILHELMS UNIVERSITÄT ZU BERLIN

By 1919, the situation had changed significantly. Europe's experience of catastrophic war and socialist revolution had swept aside orthodoxy in a variety of forms, and in Berlin, as in other cities around Europe, socialist administrators struggled with an influx of disenchanted war veterans, a scarcity of resources, the threat of hyperinflation, and political pressure from without and from within. But even in the face of all of these challenges, and less than a year after the war's end, a resolution to establish academic chairs for natural therapies at German universities was brought before the Prussian Parliament. Drafted by a committee including members of two Socialist Party factions, a Liberal, and two Center Party members, the resolution argued that the failure to provide training in physical and dietary therapies at German universities had potentially grave consequences for patients seeking treatment based upon the principles of *Naturheilkunde*.[45] The senate hoped to remedy this *de facto* hegemony of allopathic practices by creating institutional facilities to train, test, and license doctors specializing in natural therapies. The petition was unanimously ratified by the senate and quickly won support from the Social Democratic Minister for Science, Art, and Public Education, Konrad Haenisch.[46] Berlin would be the site of Germany's first contest over the implementation of the new resolution. But if, in 1919, the social, political, and economic contexts were dramatically changed, the pressure to rationalize *Naturheilkunde* had only intensified.

In autumn 1919, the medical faculty at the University of Berlin was charged with replacing the recently deceased faculty member Ludwig Brieger with a specialist in physical and dietary therapies.[47] Choosing from a short list of doctors drawn from the ranks of the Doctors' Association for Physical and Dietary Therapy (*AVpdT*), the ministry proposed Dr. Emil Klein for the position, and from the beginning, the situation was a difficult one. Not only was the medical faculty smarting over revelations in the daily press that Haenisch was trying to use the occasion of Brieger's death to create a chair for natural therapies without allocating new funds,[48] but Alfred Goldscheider, then director of the third medical clinic of the university, was already petitioning for the recently vacated seat.[49]

Equally significant was Haenisch's disclosure that he, himself, preferred natural therapies to allopathic medicine. Members of the medical faculty complained that Haenisch was trying to influence the evaluation of candidates and to insert personal preferences into a scientific process. They pointed out that the right to nominate, evaluate, and promote candidates had historically been the right and privilege of university faculties.[50] Historian Petra Werner tells us that the medical faculty's response to Klein's nomination is evidence of more general trends: faced with changing demographics, the politicization of student populations, the growing influence of social democracy, and the waning influence of educated elites in the face of mass publics after roughly 1890, many German professors engaged in defensive strategies designed to shore up the autonomy of the universities.[51] A variety of interests and assumptions influenced the search for a professor of physical and dietary therapies, and these factors help to explain the attitude of the Berlin medical faculty to the task before them. But the strategies they used to undermine Klein's candidacy, and to win back control over this space of ritual induction and exclusion, had changed dramatically from those used three decades before to indict Hermann Canitz in his trial for criminal negligence.

The faculty evaluation of Klein is an extraordinary example of the kind of boundary work that goes into creating and defending disciplinary authority, and part of what makes it special is the way that it passes over any serious consideration of Klein's research and pedagogy. Writing for the faculty, Friedrich Kraus focused not on Klein's academic record, but on educating Haenisch about the differences between academic experts and public officials, between science and speculation.[52] Kraus began his report by accusing Haenisch of injecting his personal preferences into a review process that was supposed to be both objective and organic.[53] Faculty appointments should not, in Kraus's view, be created to satisfy the desires of powerful individuals, but rather to fulfill the research needs of scientists as they pushed against the limits of scientific knowledge.[54] His report also included a warning to public officials should they fail to recognize the disciplinary division of labor. "A resolution," wrote Kraus, "is not binding when it is based upon unattainable criteria, which is undoubtedly here the case."[55] Kraus was threatening to ignore the ministry mandate if bureaucrats continued to meddle in the affairs of the medical faculty. The confrontational style that defined interwar politics was beginning to surface even in the relatively protected halls of the academy. Threatening language was only part of the strategy, though. More important was establishing boundaries between competing styles of inquiry. Kraus tried to do this by pointing to what he thought were the different methods that medical researchers and lay healers used to justify their therapies.

According to Kraus, the period after roughly 1890 had witnessed the proliferation of new "medical" models—from hydrotherapy to hypnotism, from Thure Brandt massage to movement therapy. These medical models were distinct from one another in almost every way, but they shared one key feature: they all dogmatically asserted that they alone were capable of "ensuring health and longevity."[56] Kraus avoided any direct mention of *Naturheilkunde*, and for his purposes, this omission made perfect sense. As we shall see below, Kraus wanted to argue that what laymen called *Naturheilkunde* was already a fully integrated subfield in German medical programs. Instead of attacking *Naturheilkunde* directly, then, Kraus worked to link the popular practice of natural healing to the extrascientific dogma of other "faith-based" healing traditions. He used the example of Christian Science to make his case.

The attack on Christian Science was, by 1919, a well-worn tactic. For decades, medical associations had criticized the pretensions of Christian Scientists to heal the sick, and they were not alone in their hostility. In their outspoken criticism of the war and their attempts to mobilize pacifist sentiment, their insistence on sin and purity in the etiology of sickness, Christian Scientists had antagonized not only war-minded conservatives, but also socialists committed to a scientific transformation of society and liberals convinced by a reformed religiosity. While Christian Science certainly presented an easy enough target, Kraus used it in strategic ways to highlight the differences between styles of seeing, the one rational, systematic, skeptical, and scientific, the other dogmatic, empirical, ingenuous, and unscientific. Christian Scientists, and by extension, the laymen and laywomen who practiced *Naturheilkunde*, used crude empiricism to justify their healing work. Pointing to sick patients who recovered while under their care, Christian Scientists and natural healers conflated causation with correlation.

In Kraus's view, this was not very convincing. Doctors and educated laymen well knew that, except in the worst cases, patients tended to recover from their illnesses independent of the healer's intervention. Without understanding *how* or *why* a medical condition developed the way that it did, without knowing why one treatment worked while another one did not, practitioners in these traditions took *on faith* their role in restoring a patient's health. Ultimately, this is what distinguished academic medicine from the new therapies. "The practical application of these various therapeutic systems ... [rests upon] the naïve perception that a healthy patient constitutes evidence [of therapeutic efficacy], evidence that [can be interpreted] using pure empirical observation."[57] For all of the differences between them, *Naturheilkunde* was, in this respect, just as unscientific (and dogmatic, empirical, ingenuous) as was Christian Science.

The medical faculty's refusal of lay healers and their "crude empiricism" was not meant as a rejection of what laymen called *Naturheilkunde*, and Kraus tried to highlight this by pointing to the widespread use of physical and dietary therapies in university clinics. Kraus argued that medical men had long played a role in the discovery and dissemination of physical and dietary therapies,[58] and he was able to point to widespread use of "water treatments for typhus, fresh air cures and dietary therapy for tuberculosis ... exercise programs for nervous disorders, breathing exercises for lung disease, physical therapy in treating heart conditions, dietary therapy for diabetes, kidney infections, rheumatoid arthritis, and obesity" at various university clinics.[59] To bolster claims that a new professorship was unnecessary, he argued that "no doctor leaves the university . . . without having had the opportunity to study physical therapies."[60] In important ways, this was true.[61] Kraus's evaluation was not intended to exclude physical and dietary therapies from the university. Rather, it was designed to assert disciplinary autonomy and the prerogatives of scientific experts against claims made by laymen and legislators. In the first round of these negotiations, the faculty had some success. Emil Klein was dropped from the list of candidates.[62]

Anxious to avoid a direct confrontation with the medical faculty, Haenisch called upon Weyl to submit a new list of suitable candidates, and early in 1920, Weyl suggested Franz Schönenberger, editor of Nature's Doctor, for the position.[63] While Haenisch wanted to avoid the kinds of complications that had accompanied Klein's nomination, the nomination of Schönenberger demonstrates how committed Haenisch was to implementing the senate's resolution.[64] In contrast to Kraus's evaluation of Klein, the faculty evaluation of Schönenberger showed an intimate knowledge of the candidate's research and publishing history.[65]

Schönenberger was widely respected in natural healing circles and beyond. A former school teacher, he became a natural healer in the 1890s and a licensed physician in 1898. In 1906 he replaced Gerling as editor of Nature's Doctor, and he became known as an advocate for lay healing prerogatives, a consensus-builder with interests in social hygiene, and a participant in numerous Life-reform associations. In part because of their recent failure in derailing the nominating process, the faculty had shifted away from the confrontational strategy they had used in Klein's case. But their report on Schönenberger still tried to situate his work outside the broad penumbra of regular medicine, claiming in one place that his popular two-volume The Art of Living, the Art of Healing showed that Schönenberger had "read a good many medical books, which he is able to skillfully cite when they support his opinions."[66] To say the least, this was damning with faint praise.

Schönenberger was a different kind of candidate than the faculty usually encountered, if only because he had started his medical career as a lay healer. But he was different in one other important way as well.

Unlike their own preferred candidate, Alfred Goldscheider, and unlike anyone else on the faculty, for that matter, Schönenberger had mostly practical training, and his publications were directed primarily at lay audiences. He had, of course, conducted research as part of his medical degree and had written his dissertation on the effects of sunlight on animals.[67] But his published writing consisted for the most part of short articles written for *Nature's Doctor*, manuals like *Medical Advice for Young Married People*, and handbooks like *The Art*, co-authored with his father-in-law, Wilhelm Siegert, who also happened to be a lay healer.[68] The dean of the medical faculty, clearly unimpressed, cited the candidate's "superficial and one-sided treatment of the scientific problems of physiology and pathology."[69]

This was not, however, the problem with appointing Schönenberger to the faculty position. The dean of the medical faculty had little doubt that Schönenberger was a competent clinician and a fine teacher. But the candidate simply did not have the credentials to allow the faculty to evaluate him for the position.[70] If a new faculty chair was to be created, it would have to be filled by someone who had the "right" scientific and scholarly credentials. In the view of the medical faculty, this did not include a doctor best known for his popular work and for his generalist credentials. Whatever his qualifications may have been, Schönenberger simply was not an expert.

The evaluation's praise was meant to be damning to Schönenberger's candidacy, but it also explains much about the changed status of natural therapies more generally. In 1889 we saw Dr. Wolff give testimony against Hermann Canitz not because he was a layman, but because the therapies he prescribed—moist wraps, healing oils, and immobilization—were medically heterodox. As Wolff put it, if the judge returned a not-guilty verdict, then he "might as well simply close the lecture-halls."[71] In 1889, medical men attacked natural healing as a set of marginal practices, though this was also meant to implicate the laymen who developed and used those practices. By 1920, many of those same practices were widely accepted. Now it was the lay practitioners who were targeted by those hoping to enforce disciplinary boundaries. Schönenberger may have had a medical degree and a professional license, but in his personal biography as much as in his professional choices, he had

clearly allied himself with that world of irregular practitioners.
The faculty evaluation of a third candidate, Dr. Peter Ziegelroth,
points in the same direction. According to the evaluation, Ziegelroth
was known to the scientific community largely because of his "hostility to scientifically based medicine, and his use of advertisements that
failed to meet the standards of professional honor." According to the
dean of the medical faculty, Ziegelroth "employed the most crass and
offensive language against scientific medicine and research, revealing...a
radicalism which [is] hardly to be found in any other representative of
his field." The dean did not miss the opportunity to offer his personal
impressions. He claimed that, when Ziegelroth "puts on his scientific
hat, he makes himself laughable." The faculty rejected out of hand the
Ziegelroth nomination not just because of his advocacy of lay healing
prerogatives, nor in response to his outspoken criticism of mainstream
medicine. They rejected his candidacy because he blurred the lines between medical expert and medical outsider.[72]

A look at the process leading up to the reports on Schönenberger
and Ziegelroth underlines the importance of personal biography and
background in the faculty's thinking about which candidates were legitimate contenders for the chair. When faced with the candidacy of
Schönenberger, whose research background was relatively thin, the
medical faculty balked and renewed their calls to put Alfred Goldscheider in the vacant chair. Unlike Schönenberger,[73] Goldscheider had
carefully cultivated working relations with research scientists at the
same time that he worked to promote the scientific study of physical
and dietary therapies as a cofounder of ZpdT. In their advocacy of
Goldscheider, the medical faculty signaled their readiness to integrate
physical and dietary therapies more fully into medical curricula, but
also their belief that only certain kinds of people were qualified to teach
it: medical professors with research training.

In a show of compromise, and bowing to ministry pressure to
implement the parliamentary decision, the dean of the medical college
made a couple of proposals aimed at mitigating the effects of parliament's decision. In addition to proposing the creation of new facilities
dedicated to the scientific study of physical and dietary therapies, to
be located on the outskirts of the city, he invited Schönenberger to

hold guest lectures at the university. Kraus claimed that this would give the medical faculty further opportunities to judge whether or not Schönenberger was worthy of the regular post. However, the medical faculty was not in much of a position to bargain over the matter, and Schönenberger was offered the chair of natural healing in April 1920.

Schönenberger's accession to a professorial chair in Berlin, followed in 1924 by the creation of a new chair at Jena, points to the degree to which natural healing had entered the institutional mainstream. Certainly these appointments were hotly contested by the different medical faculties. From the evaluations of Klein and Schönenberger, though, we see that medical men no longer objected to the application of physical and dietary therapies as such, but rather to the proposed candidates. How different it was, then, from 1889, when medical men indicted natural therapies simply because the therapies diverged from those accepted in university circles.[74] By all accounts, it appears that the strategy of exclusion had failed.[75]

CONCLUSION

Since its founding in 1889, the executive committee of the German League had pushed for institutions to train and license natural healers, and with the creation of nine-month courses in *Naturheilkunde* in 1892, and biannual examinations to certify the competence of students, key figures in the natural healing movement took steps in this direction.[76] This was, as they saw it, part of the work of making *Naturheilkunde* into a viable alternative to the medical mainstream, ensuring at the same time a steady supply of well-trained healers, the respectability of natural therapies, and the (relative) standardization of its practice.[77] Their efforts to bring *Naturheilkunde* into the medical mainstream found some unexpected support.

Faced with growing competition in the medical marketplace, and anxious to expand their therapeutic competence, medical men began, in the last decade of the nineteenth century, to recognize natural therapies as an uncharted route to professional advancement. Part of this had to do with the broader transformation of the medical field, which saw a growing emphasis on prevention, hygiene, and popular education.

Whatever their reasons, medical men increasingly made *Naturheilkunde* part of their therapeutic arsenal, founding professional associations like the *AVpdT* and journals like *ApdT* and *ZdpT*. If medical men turned in growing numbers to the study and practice of *Naturheilkunde*, this did not mean that they accepted the laymen and women who had pioneered those practices.

The rationalization of *Naturheilkunde* was, in part, responsible for its ongoing success. But—and here I borrow Carsten Timmermann's formulation—"rationalizing 'folk medicine'" also had a range of unintended consequences, changing the face of caregivers and negatively impacting the prospects of those who failed to produce the new kinds of credentials.[78] "Rationalizing 'folk medicine'" excluded—or at least marginalized—local knowledge and practitioners who had learned their craft outside of formal institutional frameworks. New kinds of training and licensing institutions threatened to make the new face of natural healing more male, more urban, and more prosperous. *Naturheilkunde* became part of the medical mainstream through the professionalization of its practice.

Reinhold Gerling, the quarrelsome editor of *Nature's Doctor*, commented on this state of affairs as early as 1897. Writing about the enthusiastic response to proposals for the creation of a hydropathic institute at the University of Heidelberg, Gerling claimed that the natural healing movement was signing on to a vision of knowledge production, disciplinary specialization, and expertise that would, in the end, be certain to exclude lay healers. If natural healers accepted hierarchies rooted not only in therapeutic competence but in education and accreditation, they would be helping to marginalize voices that had long asserted their independence from authorities and experts. If that happened, then "spring and mineral water [would] soon be sold at a premium in the apothecary."[79] And of course, they are.

CHAPTER FIVE

ANTI-VACCINE AGITATION, PARLIAMENTARY POLITICS, AND THE STATE IN GERMANY, 1874–1914

A t the 33rd World Health Assembly on May 8, 1980, World Health Organization (WHO) officials announced the eradication of smallpox as a naturally occurring virus. Parents, public health and government officials celebrated the news, and for the WHO, it represented a major step forward in the fight against epidemic disease. The eradication of smallpox was a major victory for global health experts who had, over a period of decades, deployed vast financial and human resources in their efforts to eradicate the disease.[1] In collaboration with governments in the developing and the developed world, officials at the WHO had taken an aggressive and sometimes controversial approach in their campaign to vaccinate hundreds of millions of at-risk young people in Asia, Africa, and South America.[2] In some cases, medical officers joined with the police and army to secure local communities and to physically restrain parents while children were vaccinated.[3] More than one observer compared the global vaccine project to a military campaign.[4] The WHO, it appeared, had won the war.

Critics of these aggressive tactics wondered, though, which war it was that the WHO was fighting. As they pointed out, the campaign against smallpox did not address the root causes of global health inequalities. Some argued that global resources would have been better deployed to ensure access to clean drinking water, hygiene infrastructure, sexual health education, and on-the-ground medical facilities.[5] It is not my goal here to evaluate the relative merits of these competing visions of public health. I do want to make clear, however, that public health initiatives like the WHO smallpox eradication program are never simply about public health: for almost two centuries, the attempt to control and ultimately eradicate smallpox has raised questions about individual and community rights, the prerogatives of medical elites and public health officers, and the scope of state power. Beginning in 1874, when compulsory vaccination was introduced in Germany, parents, activists, elected officials, and ministry bureaucracies fought over these issues. The 1874 vaccine law represented a key site in ongoing debates over medical pluralism.

This chapter traces the history of anti-vaccine agitation and shows how changing ideas about publicity shaped the strategies of both advocates and critics of the law. I show how emotion and anxiety were mobilized to overturn the law, and how this appeal to the instincts deployed scientific method and new forms of publicity to reach the widest possible audience.[6] To critics, compulsory vaccination represented a dangerous expansion of state-sponsored medicine and an abrogation of the individual's right to control his or her own body. Protest against compulsory vaccination was so powerful because it drew from multiple and overlapping communities of concern. It was driven by concerns about risk, rights, and choice.[7] Given the popularity of medical alternatives like *Naturheilkunde*, the right to make medical decisions took on an added dimension. For the many committed followers of natural healing, compulsory vaccination was just the most egregious example of an imperialistic medical establishment. Anti-vaccine activists waged an extraordinarily effective public relations campaign. Doctors were less successful. As they had so many times before, doctors failed to listen to grievances from their critics, choosing instead to attack those on the other side of the issue. This failure to address the concerns of an anxious public did little to enhance public perceptions of the medical establishment. In fact, the perception that medical authorities were aloof and unresponsive to those they served helped to galvanize a broad coalition dedicated to a free medical marketplace.

In this chapter, I use the umbrella term "anti-vaccine activist" to describe the broad and fluid coalition that came together to challenge various aspects of the 1874 vaccine law. The core of this community included the usual suspects from popular health and hygiene reform groups like the German League, the Anti-Vaccination League, and the Doctors' Association for Physical and Dietary Therapy. More interesting, though, is the way that anti-vaccine activism exceeded the boundaries of these now familiar reform movements. Anti-vaccine activism included concerned parents with little interest in *Naturheilkunde*, it included lawyers and lawmakers concerned about the exercise of unrestrained state power, and it included public-health and hygiene specialists who were not convinced of the biomedical efficacy of the national vaccine law.

Anti-vaccine agitation also casts a spotlight on fundamental tensions between popular politics, elected officials, legal institutions, and the state in Wilhelmine Germany. As we shall see, there were a number of occasions when it appeared as though parliamentary pressure and legal decisions would force the dismantling of the Wilhelmine vaccine regime. That nonelected officials—medical police, bureaucrats, and ministry officials—were able to successfully deflect these pressures tells us much about the nature of political process and power in Wilhelmine Germany. Historians have sometimes suggested that anti-vaccine sentiment was rooted in anxieties about a rapidly changing sociocultural landscape. In this chapter, I show that this is just one small part of a much more complicated story.

CONTESTING KNOWLEDGE: AUTHORITY AND EXCLUSION

Smallpox has plagued populations rich and poor, urban and rural, for thousands of years. Physical evidence shows that Ramses V died of the pox in 1157 BCE, and Shitala Mata, one of the avatars of the Hindu goddess Kali, is thought by some to have the power to either spread the disease or protect against it.[8] In the eighteenth century, at least one Bourbon monarch died of the disease, as did countless members of the higher nobility.[9] Smallpox is caused by the Variola virus, a complex and highly stable pathogen found only in human subjects.[10] The virus is nontransmissible during its incubation, which typically lasts between ten and twelve days, and transmission usually requires extended exposure to infected persons.[11]

In the initial phase of the illness,[12] infected persons may experience fever in excess of 104 Fahrenheit, rapid pulse, and head- and backaches. They also exhibit tell-tale markers of the disease: distinctive, bright red pockmarks that can be as large as two centimeters in diameter. In the second, or eruptive, phase, red pocks, mostly on the face and neck, erupt into pea-sized nodules that fill with pus. Pustules form not only on external surfaces, but also on different mucous membranes, causing pain, difficulty in breathing, and blindness, among other things. During this period, the pustules can remain localized, or they can spread to cover the face, neck, and other extremities. The third phase sees the return of fever, which drains the pustules and dries out the skin. The skin sometimes becomes so dry that it begins to rip. This can be deadly. If the infected person survives this far, the final phase begins.[13] Over the course of several days, the pustules start to heal, leaving scars in their wake. The full course of the illness lasts between four and six weeks.[14] Given the terrible nature of the illness, it is not surprising that efforts to control its spread date back centuries.

Although vaccination is widely associated with Edward Jenner's experiments of the late 1790s, different strategies to protect against smallpox infection seem to have dated back as many as 2,000 years to parts of South and East Asia.[15] The most widespread of these "traditional" practices, known as "variolation," involves harvesting lymph material from the pustule of an infected person, and then scratching a small amount of the liquid pus into the skin of the upper arm.[16] Because smallpox can only affect a person once, it was believed that inducing a mild case of the illness could produce life-long protection. Variolation, which depends on human-to-human transfer of lymph material, has its own risks. Not only is it possible to pass unrelated infections from the donor to recipient—syphilis and tetanus were commonly transmitted in this way[17]—but there is always the possibility of a violent reaction to the variolation, which can lead to the uncontrolled spread of the disease. Edward Jenner's vaccine was designed to mitigate these risks and to improve existing practices, rather than to transform those practices completely.[18]

Instead of drawing smallpox-infected pus from victims of the disease, Jenner drew vaccinia from the encrusted udder of affected cows, inserting this material into the upper arm of the small child through a series of small incisions.[19] If vaccination went well, the patient would suffer a low-grade fever, slight swelling of the affected area, and a small elevated mark where vaccine had been introduced into the body. This was called "successful" vaccination. Because cow pox typically results in a milder reaction in the recipient of the vaccine, and because it is not possible to transmit the cow pox from human to human, vaccination quickly replaced variolation in efforts to control the spread of epidemic diseases.[20] This procedure appeared to be an improvement of existing techniques, and as early as 1801, Sweden had introduced compulsory vaccination. A number of German states followed suit, with Bavaria leading the way in 1807, Baden und Kurhessen in 1815, Württemberg und Nassau in 1818, and Hanover in 1831.[21] Many thought Jenner's vaccine was a triumph of the new medical science. Others were less sanguine.

Resistance to Jenner's vaccine arose almost as soon as it was introduced, and while this reaction was a consistent feature of the European cultural, political, and medical landscape for more than a century,[22] the reasons for the opposition varied. In some cases, resistance to the vaccine had to do with dangers associated with the practice. When, for example, lymph material is harvested too late from the cow, vaccination fails entirely, leaving people who thought that they were immune to smallpox susceptible to the disease. In other cases, vaccination leads to extreme reactions, including high fever, intense cramping, pockmarks, and severe body aches. In relatively rare instances, if lymph material is contaminated with streptococcal or staphylococcal bacteria or syphilis, the vaccinee might die.[23] Problems in ensuring the quality of the lymph supply, and in ensuring an antiseptic environment for the vaccination procedure, contributed to popular suspicion of the practice.

In his exhaustive study of compulsory vaccination in Württemberg in the early nineteenth century, Eberhard Wolff has shown that, contrary to the view advanced by some contemporaries, critics of compulsory vaccination were driven less by "traditional" mentalities, superstitions, or hostility to science, progress, or state power than they were deeply concerned about the potential health risks associated with the inoculation of small children.[24] Wolff shows how parents differed from medical experts and state officials in the ways that they evaluated risk, arguing that widely publicized cases involving sickness and death as a result of vaccination contributed to anxieties about the merits of the procedure. If resistance to vaccination was, in the first part of the nineteenth century, widespread, Wolff is careful to demonstrate that it was also largely unorganized: parents protested the vaccination of their children not in their capacity as citizens, but in their role as concerned caregivers.

Anti-vaccine agitation took on a very different quality in the second half of the century. While anxiety about vaccination may have been, in the first decades of the nineteenth century, widespread, it was also largely unorganized. In the post (1848) revolutionary period, this changed. Key activists worked to channel this anxiety into organized activity. Through local associations and publicity campaigns that used statistical evidence, anti-vaccine activists mobilized popular opinion against smallpox vaccination in general, and compulsory vaccination in particular.[25] Whichever strategy they used to discredit vaccination, though, they were condemned by those on the other side of the issue. For more than a century, advocates of comprehensive vaccination accused its critics of everything from stupidity, hysteria, and uncritical superstition[26] to technophobia and fear of modernizing impulses.[27] To advocates of vaccination, resistance against a medical innovation promising human mastery of a disease seemed downright medieval.

Whatever the opinion of advocates of universal vaccination may have been, they could not deny that critics found a receptive audience. Mobilized by anti-vaccine activists like Carl Gottlob Nittinger, rates of vaccination began to fall dramatically on the eve of German unification. One commentator, a professor in Leipzig, claimed that anti-vaccine agitation "used all available tools . . . including town-hall meetings [Volksversammlungen]" and was directly responsible for declining vaccine rates, which fell 43 percent between 1868 and 1869, and then fell again in 1870.[28] In fiery speeches and dramatically titled pamphlets like Germania's Distress and her Lament for Her Children (1867), anti-vaccine activists attacked the tyranny of the state and the venality of doctors, claiming that Germany's children were victims of a "vaccine hoax."[29]

If public officials were, at first, slow to respond to the dramatically falling vaccine rates, the smallpox pandemic of the early 1870s changed the context dramatically, and in 1874, the recently formed Germany passed a national law making vaccination compulsory. Spurred to action by the 1870–1872 epidemic that killed more than 130,000 people in Prussia alone,[30] legislators enacted the recommendations of a royal scientific commission. The commission mandated that every child be vaccinated by the end of the calendar year following his or her birth[31] and be revaccinated by the end of the twelfth year of life (regardless of whether the child was attending public or private school).[32] The vaccine law contained a provision releasing parents from the mandate if vaccination threatened the health of the infant. To secure this reprieve, which could last up to one year, parents needed to file an official statement from a licensed doctor testifying to the immediate dangers posed by vaccination.[33] This would become a matter of serious contention in coming decades.

The 1874 legislation was driven by the crisis situation facing civil administrators and legislators between 1870 and 1873, when first war, and then a smallpox epidemic was responsible for significant numbers of deaths. Even in the context of this ongoing crisis, and despite reassurances that "there is no evidence that indicates that Vaccination has a negative impact on human health," the law passed by just two votes.[34] Statistics may well have been the factor that tipped the delicate balance in favor of the proposed law.[35] The role of statistics in making the state's case for compulsory vaccination is well known, and it is not my intention to rehash these arguments for and against compulsory vaccination.[36] The decades-long back-and-forth between contemporaries suggests that this is not a very productive exercise, and historical work on the subject tends to confirm this suspicion. Instead, I want to highlight the ways that different parties worked to produce scientific authority. Ultimately, it is this contest over scientific authority that explains why those on either side of the issue were so slow to concede ground.

Some historians have been particularly critical of anti-vaccine activists, suggesting that their use of evidence was based on either ignorance or cynicism.[37] The sources suggest a very different interpretation. They suggest that partisans on both sides of the issue were operating with inconclusive data—that the science itself was unstable.[38] This did not stop partisan voices from making authoritative claims. The difference between the two sides—one for and one against compulsory vaccination—was that only one of them was able to enforce its claims with the power of the state.[39] And this is essential to understanding how anti-vaccine agitation unfolded in subsequent decades. As representatives of the state ignored the increasingly diverse coalition protesting various parts of the 1874 law, critics turned to other approaches—ones that were at the time, and continue to be, widely misunderstood.

A CASCADE OF NUMBERS

The case for a national vaccine law had a number of factors in its favor, but advocates for the new law still had to support their calls for the landmark legislation. After a number of failed attempts to mobilize statistical evidence in their favor,[40] they eventually turned to the most comprehensive dataset then available: in Sweden, vaccination had been widely practiced since 1801 and made compulsory in 1816. In addition to the relative completeness of vaccination in Sweden, where vaccine rates reached close to 100 percent of the population, the kingdom had also started compiling statistical data on smallpox-related deaths as early as 1774.[41] The so-called Swedish statistics offered the chance to observe smallpox-related mortality over the course of almost a century, and to isolate the rate of change in mortality across the threshold between partial and comprehensive vaccination.

At least on the surface, graphical representation of the data seemed to provide a compelling basis for the introduction of a comprehensive plan.[42] Not only did the frequency of epidemic outbreaks decrease over the nineteenth century, but the deadliness of those outbreaks appeared to decrease as well—from a high of more than 700 deaths per 100,000 in 1778 to fewer than 100 per 100,000 as a high for the nineteenth century in 1873. Of particular significance for advocates of the proposed legislation was the timing of this shift: both morbidity from smallpox and the frequency of smallpox epidemics decreased markedly around 1801, the year that saw Sweden introduce vaccination. For advocates, at least, the Swedish statistics were thought to be sufficient to demonstrate the merits of vaccination. As the left liberal Dr. Wilhelm Löwe wrote, the merit of vaccination was "not open to discussion." In another instance, he claimed that "armed with statistics, one has proven the benefits of vaccination."[43] These were the expressions of a self-assured medical establishment confident in the support of the state. Unsurprisingly, critics of the law were less impressed.

Dr. Heinrich Böing was an unlikely critic of compulsory vaccination, and it is not clear what motivated him in his decades-long work to overturn the 1874 law. A general practitioner and vaccine officer in Ueberdingen am Rhein, Böing told readers of his 1882 *Facts of the Smallpox and Vaccine Question* that, at least in the beginning, his research had been an attempt "to convince [critics] of the rightness of the existing vaccine-protection theory." Whatever his initial intentions were, the data caused him to reevaluate his position. "It is," Böing wrote, "certainly uncomfortable to be forced, in so important a question, to change one's convictions."[44] Unlike earlier critics like Nittinger, who described vaccination in apocalyptic terms, Böing focused his attention on the statistical evidence offered by the government in defense of the law. Even Martin Kirchner, a leading member of the Imperial Vaccine Institute, conceded that Böing was no charlatan.[45]

Böing showed that, even when taken in the crudest possible terms, the Swedish data did not tell the story that advocates of the law claimed it did. The government case used graphical representation to show a dramatic decline in smallpox-related mortality around the time that vaccination was introduced in Sweden, and Böing conceded that mortality never climbed to the figure of 5,100 per million residents that it had reached in 1800. But at the same time, no clear correlation could be made between the number of incidences of smallpox mortality and the spread of vaccination. While it is true that smallpox-related deaths declined to roughly 100 per 1,000,000 between 1800 and 1810 when only 5 percent of the population was vaccinated, and reached 0 per million in 1820 when vaccination rates reached 23.7 percent, mortality from smallpox skyrocketed to 960 per million in 1874 at a time when the population was 97 percent vaccinated.[46] Advocates of compulsory vaccination wanted to argue that smallpox-related deaths had declined steadily across the nineteenth century and that this decline was the result of increasing rates of vaccination. Böing pointed out that there was no clear relationship between the two variables.[47] Böing's 1882 critique demonstrated that graphical and statistical evidence could be manipulated to convince audiences of specious arguments. He (and other vaccine critics) hoped that, once elected officials understood that the government case was based on faulty evidence, they would consider revision of compulsory vaccination.

Instead of responding to critics, defenders of compulsory vaccination tried to silence the law's detractors and claimed that its merits were beyond dispute. As framers of an 1876 resolution by the German Medical Association put it, "There are, in Science, questions that are not up for discussion," and "the vast majority of German doctors" were in agreement about the importance of vaccination.[48] Another doctor claimed that "the fundamental premise of vaccine protection is so well established that the statistics are totally superfluous: one can expect nothing more than a confirmation of the basic principle, and where this confirmation is at present absent, this can be attributed to the incompleteness [of the statistics]."[49] Ultimately this strategy—one that exaggerated the certainty of the science while minimizing concerns about its effectiveness—gave critics *more* ammunition to use against the law and its advocates.[50] One critic compared the "medico-papal vaccine-dogma" [*medizin-pabstlichen Impfdogma*] to the "ecclesiastical-papal (claim to) infallibility."[51] This was written in 1875, at the height of the *Kulturkampf*, but as we shall see, the argument would be recycled for decades.[52]

Faced with an entrenched medical establishment that appeared unwilling to listen to statistical evidence, or to consider alternative ways of managing public health, anti-vaccine activists turned to parents, the public, and *politicians* in their efforts to overturn the law. Using the language of law and rights, the free medical marketplace, personal choice, and scientific progress, they argued that the state overstepped its prerogatives in compelling parents to vaccinate. In 1900, the Imperial Office of Health noted a dramatic increase in the number of petitions calling for the repeal of the 1874 vaccine law, from 21 in 1877 to 2,951 in 1891.[53] In the ten years following the publication of the report, the number of petitions continued to grow, so much so that, by 1910, official reports and parliamentary debates rarely mentioned the cascade of petitions from interested parties. There are a variety of factors that help to account for the growth of organized anti-vaccine sentiment, but what energized opposition to the 1874 law was, to a large extent, the perception of risk.

RISK

Government testimony used to ensure passage of the 1874 law expressly stated that vaccination posed no hidden risk to the vaccinee.[54] In the decades to come, though, this clause would become an important target for anti-vaccine activism, because it was demonstrably and dramatically untrue.[55] Thousands of children suffered from more or less severe reactions to the procedure, from high-grade fever and ulcerated abscesses, to blindness and even death, and these stories consistently found their way into anti-vaccine pamphlets, the popular press, and parliamentary hearings.[56] Despite claims by high-level ministry officials, doctors' associations, and other defenders of the law, vaccination remained a dangerous procedure well into the twentieth century. Parents had every reason to be afraid.

At least three factors affected the safety of the Wilhelmine vaccine regime. For one thing, the conditions in which vaccination was administered varied dramatically. While some vaccinations were conducted by "vaccine doctors" in government-controlled facilities, others were administered by general practitioners who were uninformed about accepted protocols or who failed to properly follow established guidelines.[57] Even when lymph material was successfully extracted, processed, and administered, vaccination could result in serious symptoms. Human error was one factor affecting the security of the vaccine process, but another factor was the imperfect process of lymph extraction. Peter Frosch, for example, reported to the Ministry of Health that "the concentration of the vaccine agent" could significantly affect the intensity of the patient's reaction.[58] Lymph material was extracted in 22 vaccine institutions around Germany—the Berlin facility was attached to the municipal slaughterhouse—but it was difficult to impose effective controls on the production process.[59] For all the efforts to control vaccine production, the consistency of lymph material varied. This lack of consistency helps to explain why reactions varied so significantly from patient to patient.

Frosch noted another reason for the wide range of reactions to vaccination, even when samples from the same vaccine material were used. As he reported to the ministry, the patient's reaction depended "not just on the consistency of the material, or the operating technique of the administering doctor," but also on "the disposition of the vaccinee."[60] Peter Frosch was a member of the Institute for Infectious Diseases and a confirmed believer in both the efficacy and the safety of vaccination. But for all his assurances that vaccination was safe (one of his colleagues even suggested that it was as likely that one would die from riding the railroads as from vaccination), parents were not always satisfied that this was true.[61]

It is difficult to determine whether and to what extent fear was the motivating factor for parents who resisted vaccination. Whatever parents' reasons were, we do know what anti-vaccine activists were hoping to accomplish. They wanted to mobilize parents' anxieties to overturn the law. In monographs, pamphlets, and journals like *Nature's Doctor* and *Anti-Vaccinationist (Impfgegner)*, critics of the 1874 law used gruesome images and highly publicized stories of vaccinations gone wrong to mobilize popular sentiment.[62] Incidents of death and disfigurement may have been statistically uncommon, but for anti-vaccine activists, they represented an opportunity to illustrate the dangers of vaccination in a compelling manner. As we will see in later sections of this chapter, it was one important part of a larger strategy to shape public and political opinion.

In many instances, anti-vaccine publicity was meant to be shocking. In 1898, for example, *Nature's Doctor* reported the death of an infant from Weißwasser in Saxony. According to undocumented testimony, the child died in its mother's arms while a doctor stood by helplessly.[63] A similar report tells the story of "Walter." Born in 1889 and vaccinated that year, Walter became sick after his revaccination in 1901. "Previously the boy was hearty and hale." Just days after vaccination, though, Walter developed a massive cyst on his armpit, and soon after, he had an outbreak of sores on his face and head.[64] Walter's story ended better than the one from Weißwasser. During the second outbreak, his parents took him to a natural healer, who successfully used a Prießnitz wrapping to control the spread of the outbreaks.[65] A disturbing image of young Walter was included with the text. Covered with centimeters-long scars, ruptured pustules, and partially healed abscesses, the image suggests that death might have been a kinder fate.

Nature's Doctor reported a similar case in the next issue. According to the report, Wilhelm Schäfer of Bielefeld was "successfully" vaccinated on May 11, 1901, by a Dr. Nünninghof. Within days, a "burning abscess" appeared on the upper arm where Wilhelm had been incised. Neither Nünninghof nor any of his colleagues was able to control the outbreak, so young Wilhelm's parents took him to a natural healer, who used moist-packing to control the boy's symptoms.[66] This story, too, had a happy conclusion, unless one looked at the attached image and saw the aftereffects of "successful" vaccination. The gaping sore on his body raised questions about the effectiveness of the Wihelmine vaccine regime in a way that statistics were unable to do. Again, vaccination was directly linked to severe and debilitating illness.

It is difficult to tell how widely these reports circulated and to what extent they influenced parental decision-making. Given the degree to which the natural healing movement had penetrated German society, though, it is likely that these disturbing cases were familiar to many parents who had infants scheduled to be vaccinated or young teens who were required to be revaccinated. Ministry officials certainly seemed to think that this kind of publicity played a key role in the rise in anti-vaccine sentiment. A ministry-commissioned report from 1900 claimed that "in the press, through flyers and brochures, they fight ceaselessly against vaccination."[67] Defenders of the Wilhelmine vaccine regime thought reporting on horror stories about vaccination was disingenuous at best. In a 1914 report to parliament, Martin Kirchner suggested that the "spectacular case" was a particular genre of propaganda. Anti-vaccine activists cited a case, included a picture, detailed the lamentable outcome, and blamed vaccination.[68] The format of the reporting, though, made verification difficult, if not impossible. In his address, Kirchner went through a couple of these cases, drawn from a pamphlet written by the well-known anti-vaccine activist Hugo Wegener. Kirchner noted that Wegener cited 35,000 such incidents.[69]

If these "spectacular cases" were recognized as a particular kind of genre, one might say that defenders of the law also turned to a particular format as they responded to alleged cases of vaccine-related illnesses. Ministry-tasked defenders of the law deflected criticism by citing a range of complementary infections that might be responsible for the troubling images publicized by anti-vaccine activists. Frosch, for example, writes that complications pursuant to vaccination were the result of "improper conduct on the part of the vaccinee or the caregiver in regard to lifestyle, cleanliness (or) bandaging."[70] Kirchner made the same claim 15 years later.[71] Young vaccinees were getting sick not because the principle of vaccination was wrong, but because their immune systems were weak, or because their vaccine wounds became infected. In this view, it was the parents (or the vaccinee!) who were at fault.

Whatever Frosch, Kirchner, and others wrote in published accounts or parliamentary hearings, others in the medical community believed that claims about the safety of *vaccination* were exaggerated. A memorandum from the president of the Imperial Office of Health to the Ministry of the Interior is a case in point.[72] President Dr. Köhler wrote to tell his colleague at the ministry about the recent publication of an anti-vaccine pamphlet by Tübingen University zoology professor Friedrich Blochmann.[73] In that pamphlet, Blochmann detailed the tragic events that left his youngest son blind in one eye. Köhler gave the following summary of the pamphlet.

Blochmann had two sons, the older three years of age, the younger ten months old. The troubles began when the older boy was vaccinated. While the older boy suffered no complications from the procedure, his younger brother was not so lucky. Two weeks after his brother's vaccination, the infant had an outbreak of pustules and sores that quickly spread from the face to the ears, stomach, hands, and legs. The older boy had infected his younger brother, likely through a small cut in the neck or face region. By the time Blochmann and his wife called in a specialist, it was already too late. The infant was blind in one eye.[74]

Citing 129 other confirmed cases in which person-to-person lymph transmission resulted in dire outcomes, Blochmann called for better training for vaccine doctors. Köhler thought this was a good idea. In addition, though, he proposed "educating the relations of the vaccinee about the dangers of person-to-person lymph transmission."[75] This was an open admission that medical experts at the highest level recognized the risks associated with vaccination. Köhler's letter shows why so many parents were concerned about vaccine-related illnesses. For parents, and a sometimes outraged public, vaccination was at the *root* of these complications, whether the principle of vaccination was sound or not.[76] If an upper-middle-class family like Blochmann's could be touched by this kind of tragedy, what about other families?[77] This was a point well recognized by contemporary critics, from activists to elected officials.[78]

In fact, safety issues were a real concern for those whose living conditions complicated sound vaccination practices. The working poor, small craftsmen, and industrial workers lived in circumstances that presented particular challenges to vaccination programs. If, as the Köhler report suggested, transmission of vaccine-related bacteria could occur even through casual contact, parents needed to exercise constant vigilance to prevent the spread of infection. Vaccine wounds needed to be kept clean, wrappings needed to be changed, pustules needed to be monitored, and the young patients had to be sequestered from other children for a period of up to two weeks. How, precisely, were working parents to enforce this kind of surveillance? At the turn of the century, more than 70 percent of Prussian families of four were making 900 RM or less per year. Studies suggested that they would spend between 650 and 750 RM on subsistence.[79] For many parents laboring under these kinds of financial pressures, it would have been impossible to maintain constant vigilance over recently vaccinated children. Whatever vaccine defenders at the Ministry of Health might have thought, keeping a vaccine incision properly dressed was just one of many challenges for the working poor. They also needed to feed and house their families.

Defenders of the law acted as though vaccination occurred in a laboratory setting. But in fact, as one parliamentary critic pointed out, it occurred in overcrowded cities, where young children came in constant and uncontrolled contact with one another. It occurred in temporarily converted schoolhouses in the countryside, where dozens and even hundreds of children were vaccinated simultaneously. It occurred in

remote regions, where parents travelled long distances by foot or car-
riage to fulfill the vaccine mandate. The conditions under which the
Wilhelmine vaccine regime was administered had little to do with the
controlled environment that Kirchner and others described.[80] For concerned parents, and for those concerned with the on-the-ground administration of the Wilhelmine vaccine regime, Peter Frosch, Martin
Kirchner, and others charged with defending the 1874 law seemed to
be dangerously out of touch with the realities of vaccination practice.
This helps us to understand why so many parents worked so hard to
evade the vaccine mandate.

EVADING THE VACCINE MANDATE AND ADMINISTERING THE LAW

After the introduction of the 1874 law, government officials were
inundated by cases of noncompliance, and the problems this caused
are hard to overestimate: each year, the vaccine administration was
faced with more than 300,000 children who, for one reason or another, had escaped the vaccine mandate.[81] This created enormous demands upon low-level city, state, and ministry employees, who were
obliged to investigate, correspond with all concerned parties, write
memoranda, and make recommendations to their superiors. This was
no small task, as the case of Herr Longino from the Berlin suburb of
Steglitz makes clear.[82]

In February 1890, local medical police wrote to Longino citing his
failure to present his daughter Hedwig for vaccination. Longino replied
(by post), that Hedwig had, in fact, been vaccinated in 1889. Questions were asked and records were checked, but there was no evidence
to support Longino's claim. Finally, in February 1891, medical police
demanded that Hedwig appear for vaccination in the Berlin-Teltow facility. They gave Longino eight days to comply. In response, Longino
secured a doctor's note stating that Hedwig was too ill to undergo the
procedure. The case, though, was far from over. Five months later, in
July, Longino received another notice citing his continued failure to
comply with vaccine law. Longino's response was really too much. He
claimed that he had FORGOTTEN! The emphasis in the original report from the District President to the Minister of the Interior is some

indication of how unbelievable this was. After 17 months, involving medical police, low-level bureaucrats, and ministry officials, the case finally came to a close. Longino was fined three Marks![83] Administering the Wilhelmine vaccine regime was time-consuming, expensive, and ultimately not all that effective.[84]

The easiest thing would have been to let these cases slide quietly by. A report on the case of the "fanatical vaccine opponent" Herr Leipold, submitted to the Ministry of the Interior in March 1901, suggests why, at least from the administrative point of view, this was impossible.[85] In answering a civil complaint on his failure to comply with the 1874 law, Leipold claimed that his three children, aged 11, 9, and 7, had all survived cases of chicken pox and were therefore not subject to revaccination as per section 1 of the vaccine law. Leipold's was an attempt to stretch the letter and the spirit of the law, because exemption from the vaccine mandate was for naturally occurring *small*pox and not for the chicken pox.[86] The author of the report urged his superiors to reject the petition, arguing that defining immunity in these broad terms would ultimately be the undoing of the vaccine law: if a childhood case of the chicken pox was enough to secure an exemption from the vaccine mandate, it would become even more difficult to maintain the minimum targets necessary to preserve herd immunity. By 1900 the situation was already precarious: 2.07 percent of the population had illegally refused vaccination, and an additional 9.74 percent secured legal exemption by submitting a doctor's note declaring the child unfit for vaccination because of illness.[87] The report to the ministry concluded that this matter concerned not just Leipold, but all vaccine opponents. Conceding to their "pathological" opposition "would strengthen the resolve not just of Leipold but of all vaccine opponents."[88]

These claims were supported by recent cases of systemic noncompliance. In 1898, for example, 1,000 parents in Hanover were fined for failure to comply with the 1874 law, and this created all sorts of administrative and legal problems, tying up court officials, police clerks, ministry subalterns, and others.[89] By the 1890s at the very latest, anti-vaccine activists were using pamphlets and publications to educate parents about how to use provisions of the law to evade the vaccine mandate.[90] Parents were instructed to delay vaccination for as long as possible, to secure doctors' notes testifying that their children were too sick to undergo the procedure, to respond to bureaucratic inquiries at the latest possible date, and to use whatever legal means possible to postpone the procedure. This may seem like a quixotic endeavor, but parents could, in this way, easily delay vaccination for up to two years without ever breaking the law, or resorting to an administrative appeals process.[91]

When parents had exhausted these legal options, a 1902 pamphlet suggested that they "apply to the provincial governor . . . or, if necessary, to the Minister of Culture who is, for such matters, the highest authority." It is not clear whether the pamphlet's author expected this appeal process to work for parents. As he noted, though, "The appeal is free *and lasts for a relatively long time.*"[92] Whether or not parents could indefinitely evade the vaccine mandate, the 1902 pamphlet offers an insight into evolving debates over the 1874 law. Critics of the law were systematically trying to overload the Wilhelmine Vaccine Administration. Decades of anti-vaccine agitation had made the administration of the Wilhelmine Vaccine Regime increasingly difficult, and by the first decade of the twentieth century, it was becoming clear that something needed to be done to achieve a workable solution.

This was all part of a broader legal problem, though. When the vaccine law passed in 1874, a bare majority (141–140) voted that there would be no national policy governing enforcement.[93] This meant that the vaccine law was administered differently across the country: towns and districts and provincial governments each had an extraordinary amount of discretion in the administration of the 1874 law. In Munich and Düsseldorf, for example, decisions taken by Provincial High Courts in 1905 and 1906 stated that the attempt to coerce compliance with the law through undue financial pressure—let alone, physical coercion—was beyond the authority of police and bureaucratic authorities.[94] The *Deutsche Tageszeitung* reported that the Hanover Police Department took a similar position: the police commissioner stated that his department would issue only one fine for noncompliance. In Hanover, parents would pay just three Marks for refusing to vaccinate their children.[95] In these places, the opportunity costs for noncompliance were remarkably low. Prussia, by way of contrast, determined that police officials had "not only a right but a duty" to enforce the vaccine mandate. If this included repeated fines, or even pulling children out of their homes, the police were in their rights to do so.[96]

If Germany's federal system contributed to the perception that the law was being applied in a capricious manner, human factors also led to uneven enforcement. After all, the officials administering the law *themselves* had strong feelings, not just about the vaccine law, but also about medical pluralism in general. When, for example, the Provincial High Court in Hamm empowered police to use a range of coercive powers to compel compliance with the vaccine law, their decision was reversed when they were on summer recess.[97] As the *Deutsche Tageszeitung* told readers, decisions on vaccination-law enforcement that were given down from provincial high courts varied. Some high courts stated their intention of using repeated fines or even physical coercion to compel compliance with the law, while others took the opposite approach to noncompliance. In some cases, one and the same court would hand down conflicting opinions. As the *Deutsche Tageszeitung* noted, "[It had] yet to be established whether repeated fines on the grounds of vaccine refusal [were] legally justified."[98] When it came to the state's ability to compel compliance with the law, there was no clear mandate. One thing, however, was clear enough: this "situation of legal uncertainty" was "unsustainable."[99]

THE PARLIAMENTARY STRATEGY

For decades, anti-vaccine activists had tried to move the government position through statistical data, case reports on the harmful effects of vaccination, and impassioned pleas by opponents of the law. Official efforts to shut down debate, to coerce parents, to demonize critics, and to operate through extra-legal measures ultimately helped to energize the opposition. Realizing that ministry officials and public health experts were not going to move on the issues, anti-vaccine activists turned to other channels. Intransigence on the government side of the vaccine debate helped to create a *political* campaign to overturn the law.

An explicitly political strategy was already in place for the 1893 elections, when an editor at *Nature's Doctor* informed readers that they could count on the support of 86 Reichstag members in their efforts to overturn the 1874 law. This was a fairly extraordinary number, representing 22 percent of all parliamentary members. Perhaps even more impressive was their support within particular parties. In the 1893 legislative cycle, 39 of the 48 Social Democratic members supported the anti-vaccine cause, 14 of 101 Center Party members did, and ten members of the various anti-Semitic parties.[100] The 1898 election saw anti-vaccine activists—led by the Anti-Vaccination League and the German League for Natural Healing—expand their activities significantly. With costs underwritten by the German League, "trusted activists" were sent to election assemblies in the "most diverse electoral districts" across Germany to find out what candidates thought about vaccination and about the 1874 law. They wanted to make candidates go on record about the rights and duties of individuals, the limits of state power, and their views on vaccination.

The move into electoral politics was, at its core, a strategic decision, because while medical doctors were heavily represented in the various government ministries charged with defending the vaccine law, they made up only a tiny fraction of parliamentary representatives.[101] Anti-vaccine activists had grown frustrated with the "reactionary" minister of health and with the general intransigence of public health bureaucrats,[102] so they sought to drive political opinion through democratic processes. With representatives in more than 200 electoral districts, anti-vaccine activists effectively turned the 1874 law into an electoral issue.[103] Mobilizing popular opinion to press a political campaign turned out to be far more effective than focusing solely on the biomedical conflict. In 1898, editors at Nature's Doctor told readers that, in the coming election cycle, they would have "supporters in all parties, and in most cases, these [elected officials] describe themselves as 'committed vaccine opponents' who promise to approach the issue in the manner of [the Anti-Vaccination League]."[104]

Fifteen years later, the effectiveness of this strategy was impossible to deny, and at least one parliamentary member claimed that the influence of anti-vaccine activists was too strong. Otto Fischbeck, a member of the Freisinnige Volkspartei, warned in 1914, "The situation has gone so far that in particular districts in the electoral campaign, the question is asked: 'how do you stand on the vaccine question?'" For some citizens, vaccination was becoming the *decisive* electoral issue.[105] The ability of anti-vaccine activists to affect parliamentary politics was the product of a decades-long project to mobilize concerned parents, scientific skeptics, and citizens concerned with individual rights and state intrusion.

If anti-vaccine activists were concerned about the dangers of vaccination and the power of the medical establishment, parliamentary opposition to the law was to a large extent a reaction to the unconstrained exercise of power by state ministries. In parliamentary debates spanning more than a decade, elected officials focused their attention on the state's use of coercion to compel compliance with the 1874 law, and on the efforts to curtail access to the free medical marketplace. In parliamentary hearings in 1898, 1902, 1907, 1911, and 1914, speakers from the Center and Social Democratic parties in particular consistently raised issues of state coercion in the administration of the vaccine law. It is not surprising that members of the Center and the Social Democratic Party would advocate for freedom of conscience and freedom from state intrusion—after all, constituencies of each party had been, if in different ways, proscribed by the central state in the 1870s and 1880s.[106] Social Democrat Paul Reißhaus, for example, noted that attempts to compel parents to vaccinate their children were in clear violation of "the spirit of the vaccine law, which envisioned relatively minor monetary penalties."[107] It was time, he argued, to standardize the administration of the 1874 law by determining whether or not the state had the power to compel vaccination "without parental consent."[108] Reißhaus was himself skeptical of vaccination and therefore would have been at odds with many of his parliamentary colleagues. But as session reporter Gustav Gäbel (German Social Reform Party—Anti-Semite) stated, "Everyone agreed that the existing vaccine law and the corresponding coercion [is seen as] an 'unjustified intrusion into family law' by the broadest section of the public."[109] Whatever their opinion of vaccination as such, parliamentary representatives understood that the law was widely perceived as coercive and capricious.

Anti-vaccine activists hoped that parliamentary representation would change the terms of the debate, but it became clear that ministry representatives could as easily ignore parliament as they could the public. As early as 1898, the state had promised a review of the 1874 law.

Responding to public and parliamentary pressure, Prussian Minister of State Graf von Posadowsky told a parliamentary commission that the relevant ministries would review existing vaccine procedures and recommend improvements to safety protocols.[110] Despite these assurances, parliamentary members heard nothing further from Posadowsky. A 1902 petition introduced by Social Democrats Friedrich Thiele and Paul Reißhaus was sent to the chancellor with similar results. The philologist and Center Party Member Maximilian Pfeiffer thought that ministries were colluding to simply bury the issue. After all, bureaucratic tenures were unlimited, unlike those of elected officials. Electoral continuity did seem to be a problem for creating a stable parliamentary opposition to the Wilhelmine Vaccine Regime: Pfeiffer claimed that colleagues in each new legislative period had to be educated about earlier initiatives to review the law.[111]

Passive resistance and foot-dragging by the relevant ministries effectively derailed reform efforts initiated by democratically elected representatives of the German people, and this helps to explain why parliamentary debates in 1902, 1911, and 1914 were so remarkably similar. In each of these cases, parliamentary critics of the 1874 law were forced to rehearse the same arguments, only to be frustrated by an entrenched and intransigent bureaucracy. Pfeiffer promised that he and his colleagues would continue to bring the matter to the parliamentary floor as many times as was necessary to get a full review of the law. He and his elected colleagues had a responsibility to do this, because they were the voice for the "hundreds of thousands" of voices that the government refused to hear.[112]

The problem, of course, was that the German parliament had little ability to impose its will on the government without using its control over the Imperial purse strings as leverage, and this was a power and privilege that parties across the political spectrum used only in extraordinary circumstances.[113] Questions of medical pluralism, the regulation of the medical marketplace, and the administration of the Wilhelmine Vaccine Regime were decisive issues for members of the voting public, and they were clearly important to some parliamentary members as well. Significant parliamentary minorities actively opposed the capricious administration of the vaccine regime, just as they had worked to ensure ongoing access to the free medical marketplace. Popular and parliamentary support, though, was not enough to change the course of government policy.

Anger over police coercion was a consistent feature of parliamentary debates, anti-vaccine pamphlets, and public meetings at least until the First World War, but when parliamentary members attacked the coercive and capricious actions of police and bureaucratic authorities, they were also protesting the unrestrained exercise of state authority. Reißhaus and Thiele in 1902, and Pfeiffer and Fassbender in 1911, were protesting not just the coercion of parents, but also the capricious way that the parliament and the judiciary were handled by representatives of the state. As Pfeiffer put it, it was time for the chancellor to treat petitions introduced by key parliamentary voting blocks in a serious way, rather than "as fodder for the waste-paper basket."[114] In their repeated challenges to the 1874 law, parliamentary representatives were engaged in a battle that went beyond the issue of vaccination: they were taking on an unresponsive and entrenched bureaucracy.

CONCLUSION: EVALUATING ANTI-VACCINE AGITATION

For generations, defenders of vaccination continued to call its critics "reckless," "criminal," "dangerous," and "foolish."[115] Even in the face of contradictory evidence, they continued to insist that vaccination was safe and effective. They continued to claim that medical opinion was unanimous in its support for vaccination. And they claimed that medical science stood above personal, professional, and party interests. Defenders of the 1874 law, from Wilhelm Löwe in the 1870s to Martin Kirchner, were convinced that their critics were reactionaries who rejected science and progress. As the National Liberal Friedrich Endemann told his parliamentary colleagues in 1902, "If you subordinate medical science to (lay opinion), then there is absolutely no need for Science."[116] In Endemann's view, experts should be the ones making choices about public health, not parents.

Historians and educated laypersons have too often taken the rhetoric of doctors' associations and state-appointed defenders of the vaccine law at face value. They have assumed that, whatever critics of the law may have claimed, they really were a force of reaction in Wilhelmine Germany. Susan Pedersen's review of Nadja Durbach's excellent book illustrates the interpretive consequences of this deeply ideological way of seeing.[117] In a review clearly driven by concerns about the present political climate in the United States in general, and falling rates of MMR vaccination in England and the United States in particular, Pedersen suggests that maybe historians have gone too far in their effort to give voice to historical "losers" like the anti-vaccine activists. Pedersen is particularly exasperated with what she calls, rather clumsily, "anti-condescensionism," that Thompsonian concern with "not just the poor stockinger or Luddite but the Homeopath and the spiritualist, the dress reformer and now, the anti-vaccinationist."[118] Pedersen is frustrated by these undereducated types who feel compelled to make themselves heard, despite their questionable pedigrees. The historical problem (but one that seems not to concern Pedersen), is that this was *not* a class-structured debate, nor was it about access to educational resources. Anti-vaccine activists opposed vaccination because there was (and continues to be) compelling evidence that there are healthy alternatives to compulsory campaigns like the one initiated in Germany in 1874.

When it comes to compulsory vaccination, historians have had a hard time recognizing that healthy alternatives were in fact possible, and this difficulty can be explained by one insurmountable fact: roughly 100 years after the smallpox campaign began in Germany, the disease was eradicated as a naturally occurring phenomenon. The *bio-medical* fact of smallpox eradication displaces the *historical* facts that defined the debate over compulsory vaccination in Wilhelmine Germany: the WHO's success in eradicating smallpox seems to be evidence that anti-vaccine activists were wrong, while vaccine advocates were correct.

Andreas Holger Maehle goes one step farther, when he claims that the German anti-vaccination movement was a complete failure, not just because of the success of the WHO campaign, but because anti-vaccine activists failed in their efforts to win a revision or even a review of the 1874 law. If one evaluates anti-vaccine agitation by its success in overturning the 1874 law, as Maehle does, then it was, indeed, a failure.[120] But as we shall see, Maehle's interpretation ultimately obscures more than it explains. Were anti-vaccine activists reactionaries, as Pedersen suggests? Were their efforts a "failure," as Maehle argues? These are two different, if related, questions. It is worth thinking about what contemporary critics of the vaccine law had to say about the forces of "reaction" and "progress."

In a 1902 parliamentary hearing, for example, the Social Democrat Friedrich Thiele claimed that doctors were interested less in public health than they were in preserving their professional rights and privileges. The vaccine debate, he said, is not about "the opposition between science and laity," but between "the untainted human understanding and a medical papistry."[121] By supporting the "vaccine dogma," by refusing to support a full review of the vaccine law, in demonizing their critics, and in ignoring popular opinion and parliamentary voices, Thiele thought that state-sponsored medicine was inhibiting progress. After all, as another Social Democrat reminded parliamentary members in 1914, "Medical science . . . has thrown overboard many principles that they defended vigorously just 50 or even 30 years ago."[122] Critics of the 1874 law—many of them defenders of medical pluralism and a free medical marketplace—had long been attacked by the medical establishment for being anti-scientific and reactionary. Responding to the "extraordinarily reactionary point of view" of one of his parliamentary colleagues, the anti-Semite Max Liebermann von Sonnenberg claimed it was, in fact, defenders of the 1874 law who took a dim view of science's promise. "I think more highly of science than [Dr. Müller—National Liberal] does. He wants to forbid these chambers to debate the vaccine question for now and the future." For Müller, the matter was settled. "I, on the other hand, believe that science never stands still."[123] Critics of the 1874 law did not reject science. They wanted *better* science.

When it comes to the 1874 vaccine law, deciding who was a progressive and who was a reactionary is no easy task. Perhaps it is the wrong way of approaching the issue. The task is no easier when it comes to evaluating Maehle's claim that the German anti-vaccine campaign was a complete failure. What, in this context, does failure really mean? Not only did social hygiene, prevention, and public education gain ground against bacteriological explanations in the Wilhelmine era, but these ways of thinking about the body helped to shape the language used to talk about health. Nor should one assume that these kinds of arguments simply disappeared as a result of medical advances during the two World Wars. Epidemic outbreaks in 1916, for example, cast further doubt on the already questionable claim that vaccination was the best way to provide security against smallpox.[124] Anti-vaccine activists also continued to find a receptive audience both in civil society and parliament: 1927, for example, saw further efforts to repeal the law debated on the floor of the Reichstag.[125]

The effectiveness of anti-vaccine activism, then, is far more difficult to measure than Maehle's account suggests. Anti-vaccine activism shaped the way that many Germans perceived the medical establishment and the ways that elected officials engaged with the various organs of state. Critics of compulsory vaccination were also calling for a new biomedical regime, one that addressed underlying problems of public health and hygiene, rather than relying on so-called silver bullets and patchwork remedies.[126] As one author in *Nature's Doctor* put it, better public health would be achieved "through better living conditions, the creation of healthier and cheaper housing and bathing facilities."[127] And as we know from earlier chapters, Anti-vaccine activists in Germany were proposing a social reorganization that included better public health and better health education. They were suggesting that social inequality played a key role in determining life opportunities, and that physical fitness, access to quality public housing, green space, clean air, and water might be better ways of controlling infectious diseases than the quick fix offered by vaccination.

The society they proposed was more egalitarian in other ways too. It was one that allowed laymen and laywomen to speak, if not equally, then at least publicly, with medical and other professional experts, where they could contest the statistics and the epidemiology, the prevention and the cure. And as historians like Andreas Daum, Cornelia Regin, and Carsten Timmermann have shown, this contest over authority and access helped to shape the ways that medicine was practiced, public health was imagined, and politics was negotiated in Wilhelmine Germany. In their calls to revisit and revise the 1874 law, in their demands for the introduction of a conscience clause, parliamentary critics of compulsory vaccination called for a government that responded to the voices of the people. In their efforts to create an impartial commission to evaluate the vaccine law, they hoped for a better science refined in a free-medical marketplace. Anti-vaccine activism was as much about hope for a better future as it was about anxieties about the present. As I suggested at the outset, this story is far more complicated than we may sometimes assume.

CONCLUSION
Rethinking Medicine and Modernity:
Popular Medicine in Practice

*W*e *Lived for the Body* explores how *Naturheilkunde* evolved, survived, and thrived over a period of roughly 120 years and makes up part of an ongoing effort to rethink "Wilhelminism and its Legacies." This study also attempts to recapture "futures past"—the possible futures imagined by Wilhelmine reformers. In the chapters on the nineteenth century roots of *Naturheilkunde* and on nature in the Wilhelmine era, I show how the practice of popular medicine shaped German ideas about nature, and how these ideas in turn changed the way natural healers thought about health and the body. Since the early nineteenth century, nature was thought to be a model for "the cure." By the end of the century, natural healers and lifestyle entrepreneurs began to imagine nature as a model for not only healing but also healthful living. As *Naturheilkunde* evolved through the nineteenth century, it became a point of contact between a constellation of so-called Life-reform movements that were concerned with everything from fashion and leisure to housing policy and public hygiene. Historians have increasingly recognized that this constellation of reform movements played an important role in the Wilhelmine public sphere, driving popular opinion and even generating local, regional, and national political engagement.

There were dozens of other organizations that were concerned with "reform" during the period between 1890 and 1918, and these organizations addressed issues large and small. Some (e.g., the German Navy League, the Pan-German League, and the German Society for Public

Health) exerted tremendous influence on popular opinion and policy directions. Others catered to just a few local members. The natural healing movement was, in this sense, just one among the myriad reform associations that populated the Wilhelmine landscape. But as I hope to have shown, it was also something more than just one among many movements: it played a central role in public and private lives. Natural healers laid hands on their patients; lifestyle entrepreneurs sold food products, self-help books, clothing, and bathing implements to Germans concerned with health and wellness; and natural healing associations provided social networks, bathing and sport facilities, educational outlets, and an introduction to local political activism. It was possible to participate in the movement as a dedicated member or a party activist, but it was also possible to be an occasional observer or even an outsider who just went to the baths or bought products associated with healing and wellness. Even for those who had little sympathy for the natural healing movement (for example, the members of the Women's Association for the Advancement of Morality, whom we encountered in chapter 2), the principles and practices of the natural healing movement were familiar ones. And this is why, in my view, the natural healing movement was so successful: it was able to shape the Wilhelmine experience in part because it touched individual lives in casual ways (e.g., in bathing facilities that were enjoyed by millions) and in transformative ones. In the process, the natural healing movement helped to define the ways that Wilhelmine Germans thought about nature, health, individual bodies, and bodies social.

In the second part of this book, I explored some of the particular challenges that faced *Naturheilkunde* in the late nineteenth and early twentieth centuries and how the movement survived those challenges. As German medical associations tried to marginalize natural healing, the German League was joined by unlikely allies who claimed, for a variety of reasons, that natural healers were legitimate players in the free medical marketplace. Some of these allies were simply defending the rule of law and expressed no particular affinities for *Naturheilkunde* as such. Others thought that a competitive medical marketplace was important to ensure the continued evolution of medicine in its theory and practice. In this view, *Naturheilkunde* and "university medicine" complemented each another, with each pushing the other to provide better care. On the surface, those citing the rule of law and those concerned with better medicine seem to have little in common. Both positions, though, point to one important fact: medical associations were unable to sell their story to the public, or to convince enough people—police officials, legislators, newspaper editors, patients, consumers—that *Naturheilkunde* was marginal medicine.

Part of the reason for the inability of "official medicine" to prevail was its inept public relations. But there is another, more important, reason: doctors' associations were unable to convince the public that *Naturheilkunde* was marginal *because it was not, in fact, marginal.* We have seen how ubiquitous and pervasive the "back-to-nature" movement had become in Germans' daily lives and how its appeal cut across political and confessional lines. This is not to say that Germans across the board sympathized with the natural healing movement. Many, in fact, mocked natural healers for their superstitious ways and outmoded beliefs. In the end, though, doctors' associations were unable to convince the public that *Naturheilkunde* was dangerous or that natural healers were quacks. The ongoing failure to close down the free medical marketplace is one important indication of this.

It turns out that it is possible to read the survival story of *Naturheilkunde* in the nineteenth and early twentieth centuries as a triumphal narrative: despite the attempts to marginalize the movement, consumers still bought reform products and lifestyle entrepreneurs became famous, open-air sun parks opened in the hundreds, the German League expanded its membership, and the medical marketplace remained remarkably open. However, this triumph was costly. As enterprising young doctors integrated *Naturheilkunde* into their therapeutic arsenal, as institutes for hydrotherapy and university chairs were created, some of the qualities that had made *Naturheilkunde* distinctive began to change. For one thing, medical men were never willing to accept lay healers as their equals, even as they began to use natural therapies in a more systematic way. As natural therapies were institutionalized in medical books and university lecture halls, the lay healers who had played the key role in developing natural therapies were pushed toward the margins of the medical marketplace. And it was not just the face of the natural healer that was transformed through the professionalization of *Naturheilkunde's* practice. As natural therapies were integrated into an eclectic approach to health care, the holistic principles that made *Naturheilkunde* distinctive were slowly compromised. For much of the nineteenth century, natural healers had argued that nature could be a model not just for curing the sick, but also for healthful living. In the hands of allopathic doctors, *Naturheilkunde* became, once again, more about therapies than everyday practices.

The natural healing movement is a fascinating chapter in the Wilhelmine story, but many readers will want to know: What came next? Was natural healing eventually superseded by university medicine? Did therapeutic, technological, and pharmaceutical advances prove, once and for all, that university-trained doctors had been right all along in asserting the superiority of their theory and practice?[1]

NATURHEILKUNDE IN THE "THREE GERMANYS": A SHORT EPILOGUE

In 1939, Chief Medical Officer of the Nazi Regime Gerhard Wagner claimed that it was not possible for the state "to create the wondrous unity of a people." The state, claimed Wagner, "can only smooth the path." The people, for their part, "must travel the road themselves."[2] Under his direction, the natural healing movement was promised a new place in the sun, with state support for teaching, training, research, and hospitals. The National Socialist Party appeared ready and willing to "smooth the path" for the natural healing movement. And the historical record suggests that the organized followers of *Naturheilkunde* were prepared to "travel the road themselves."

Licensed practitioners of *Naturheilkunde* seemed particularly eager to sign on to the National Socialist project. In March 1933, the Doctors' Association for Natural Healing-South voted unanimously to join the National Socialist Doctors' League, and the South Group of the Doctors' Association for Physical and Dietary Therapy joined the National Socialist working group for medicine in early 1934. Paul Schirrmeister joined the National Socialist Party early on, as did Karl Strunckmann of the Doctors' Association for Natural Healing. In 1934, the Johannstädter Hospital in Dresden was renamed for Ru-

dolf Heß, who was a champion of *Naturheilkunde*. Alfred Brauchle—
one of Schönenberger's students—was appointed to head the natural
healing clinic. Editors at *Nature's Doctor* also got on board. In 1933,
they expressed their confidence that the German League would find
greater recognition under the new regime.[3]

It is hard to tell how much of this was ideological and how much
was opportunistic. After all, Schirrmeister, Brauchle, Strunckmann,
and others had all supported the Social Democratic Minister Konrad
Haenisch in his efforts to create new chairs for health and healing at
German universities at the beginning of the Republic. Like Haenisch
before him, Wagner promised to be a champion for the natural healing movement. Whatever the motivation may have been, the German
League joined the newly created National Socialist Working Group for
a *Neue Deutsche Heilkunde* in 1935. The working group was supposed
to chart a new way forward for German medicine, bringing together
indigenous healing traditions like *Naturheilkunde*, *Homöopathie*, and
Biologische Medizin with allopathic medicine. Under the aegis of the
Neue Deutsche Heilkunde, diverse healing traditions would be formally
equal, with doctors, healers, and researchers working together regardless of training or tradition, to find practical health care solutions to
pressing social and medical problems. In medicine, as in so much else,
it appears that the Nazis had created something radically new out of
fragments of the past.[4]

The story, it turns out, was more complicated than it appeared. The
Neue Deutsche Heilkunde may at first have seemed to be everything that
the German League could have hoped for, creating parity between the diverse healing traditions and promising new institutional resources for the
dissemination of *Naturheilkunde*. But these concessions came at a price.
For one thing, Wagner demanded that in the interest of public health,
the different healing traditions put aside the principles that brought
them into conflict with one another. This meant, among other things,
that the German League would have to put aside many of the principles
that distinguished *Naturheilkunde* from the other healing traditions in
the first place —its call for a nonpharmaceutical medicine, its criticism of
vaccination, and its rejection of localized diagnostic methods.[5]

Wagner promised many things in exchange for these concessions, but he was also fighting battles of his own against powerfully entrenched interest groups, and by the late 1930s the ideological work of creating a distinctively German healing tradition was subordinated to the practical work of military preparedness. With the possibility of war looming, no one wanted to antagonize the doctors who would care for men in uniform, or who would take charge of public health on the home front. It turns out that, for all the rhetoric of a *Volksgemeinschaft*, of *Gleichschaltung*, of ideological uniformity and the like, Nazi Germany was shot through with the same kinds of institutional, professional, and administrative tensions that earlier regimes had faced. While some of these tensions were erased through political and racial violence, others—for example, the conflict between lay healers and licensed doctors, between *Naturheilkunde* and academic medicine—were more persistent, transcending, as they did, political, confessional, and "racial" categories. In any event, the National Socialist Working Group for a *Neue Deutsche Heilkunde* was dismantled in January 1937, just months after it was created.[6] The Nazi regime, which had promised so much to the organized followers of *Naturheilkunde*, proved to be their undoing. In this way, too, the German League imperfectly reflects the German story more generally.

The histories of organized *Naturheilkunde* took two very different paths in postwar Germany. In the German Democratic Republic, party functionaries and propagandists thought that the allegedly romantic, antiscientific, and anti-urban ideology associated with *Lebensreform* in general, and *Naturheilkunde* in particular, had played a role in the smoke-and-mirrors mystification that had paved the way for the triumph of "fascism." *Naturheilkunde* became, in the hands of party ideologues, one part of a broader project of de-Nazification— one that was designed to liberate the GDR from Germany's recent past, as much as it was to tie the capitalist West to the National Socialist regime. At least in their efforts to control organized *NaturheilkundeBad break: Natur/heil/kunde*, the GDR was extraordinarily effective: in 1989, there were only *twelve practitioners* specializing in natural therapies.[7] While it is impossible to say for certain how, and to what extent, natural healing and natural lifestyles continued to be part of the East German experience, it is clear that the institutional practice of *Naturheilkunde* was stripped out of the public health apparatus. The situation was very different in the Federal Republic, where some 35,000 doctors specialized (or had subspecialties) in natural therapies.[8] The postwar West saw the popularity of natural therapies, medicines, and consumer products grow, and that popularity continues to be evident in Germany's medical marketplace. In the West, though, consumers and practitioners alike have tended to filter the social criticism out of the practice of alternative medicine, preferring instead to attend to the individual body. In either case, the ways that Germans East and West thought about health and the body, consumption and physical restraint, have much to tell us about the twin trajectories of a divided Germany.[9]

The story of organized *Naturheilkunde* is filled with irony. A holistic medical tradition that had a tremendous popular following, *Naturheilkunde* lost some of its distinctive qualities just as it was integrated into the medical establishment. A healing ideology that stressed the transformative possibilities of individual practices, *Naturheilkunde* was used to justify race-purity laws that denied agency to individual actors. A health and hygiene movement that aimed to transform the national conversation about public health, *Naturheilkunde* wound up mostly transforming localities, where it pushed cities to build sport and bathing facilities, induced hospitals to create clinics for *Naturheilkunde*, and initiated public-private partnerships to reform urban land use. But ultimately the organized followers of *Naturheilkunde* wanted to change the ways that people thought about health and the body, and they may have done this. In the end, it was in the areas of leisure and lifestyle, of unconscious practices and preferences, that *Naturheilkunde* left its enduring mark on the ways that many Germans thought, and continue to think, about nature, health, and the body.

NOTES

INTRODUCTION

1. Some of this "doubt" is manufactured for political and economic purposes. See the excellent monograph by Naomi Oreskes and Erik Conway, *Merchants of Doubt: How a Handful of Scientists Obscured the Truth on Issues from Tobacco Smoke to Global Warming* (New York: Bloomsbury, 2010).

2. Some notable exceptions include Wolfgang Krabbe, *Gesellschaftsveränderung durch Lebensreform: Strukturmerkmale einer sozialreformerischen Bewegung im Deutschland der Industrialisierungsperiode* (Göttingen: Vandenhoeck und Ruprecht, 1974); Karl Eduard Rothschuh, *Naturheilbewegung, Reformbewegung, Alternativbewegung* (Stuttgart: Hippokrates Verlag,1983); Ulrich Linse, *Barfüssige Propheten. Erlöser der zwanziger Jahre* (Berlin: Siedler Verlag, 1983) and his *Ökopax und Anarchie: eine Geschichte der ökologischen Bewegungen in Deutschland* (München: Deutscher Taschenbuch Verlag, 1986).

3. Eva Barlösius, *Naturgemässe Lebensführung: zur Geschichte der Lebensreform um die Jahrhundertwende* (Frankfurt: Campus Verlag, 1997), 239–45; Florentine Fritzen, *Gesünder Leben: Die Lebensreformbewegung im 20 Jahrhundert* (Stuttgart: Franz Steiner Verlag, 2006), 36; Krabbe, 12–13.

4. David Blackbourn and Geoff Eley, *The Peculiarities of German History: Bourgeois Society and Politics in Nineteenth-Century Germany* (New York: Oxford University Press, 1984); Geoff Eley and James Retallack eds., *Wilhelminism and Its Legacies: German Modernities, Imperialism, and the Meanings of Reform, 1890–1930* (New York: Berghahn Books, 2003); Kevin Repp, *Reformers, Critics, and the Paths of German Modernity: Anti-politics and the Search for Alternatives, 1890–1914* (Cambridge, MA: Harvard University Press, 2000); Thomas Rohkrämer, *Eine andere Moderne: Zivilisationskritik, Natur und Technik in Deutschland, 1880–1930* (Paderborn: Schöningh Verlag, 1999); John Williams, *Turning to Nature in Germany: Hiking, Nudism, and Conservation, 1900–1930* (Stanford: Stanford University Press, 2007).

5. This work began in earnest with Cornelia Regin's path-breaking study, though earlier studies by Wolfgang Krabbe and Ulrich Linse certainly set the tone for future research. Cornelia Regin, *Selbsthilfe und Gesundheitspolitik. Die Naturheilbewegung im Kaiserreich, 1889–1914* (Stuttgart: Franz Steiner Verlag, 1995).

6. The first of these was the *"Ansbacher Verein,"* founded by the gymnasium teacher E. F. C. Oertel. The group soon changed its name to *"Hydropathischer Hauptverein,"* which saw sister organizations founded in Berlin, Dresden, Eisenach, Kassel, Lübeck, and elsewhere in the middle and later 1830s. Regin (1995), 31.

7. After 1900, the German League of Natural Lifestyle and Healing Associations (*Deutscher Bund der Vereine für naturgemäße Lebens- und Heilweise*). Regin (1995), 45. Hereafter I refer to this umbrella organization as "The German League."

8. Regin (1995), 49–51.

9. Kai Buchholz et al., eds., *Die Lebensreform: Entwürfe zur Neugestaltung von Leben und Kunst um 1900* (Two Volumes: Darmstadt: Institut Mathildenhöhe–Häusser, 2001).

10. Fritzen, 176.

11. Williams, 2–3.

12. Hugo Höppener, Gusto Gräser, Wilhelm Bölsche, Karl May, and Magnus Hirschfeld were just a few of the important figures involved in the *Lebensreform* movement.

13. Rohkrämer, 1999.

14. Fritzen, 2006; Michael Hau, *The Cult of Health and Beauty in Germany: A Social History, 1890–1930* (Chicago: University of Chicago Press, 2003); Uwe Heyll, *Wasser, Fasten, Luft und Licht. Die Geschichte der Naturheilkunde in Deutschland* (Frankfurt: Campus, 2007); Robert Jütte, *Geschichte der alternativen Medizin: von der Volksmedizin zu den unkonventionellen Therapien von Heute* (Munich: C. H. Beck, 1996); Regin, 1995; Carsten Timmermann, "Rationalizing 'Folk Medicine' in Interwar Germany: Faith, Business, and Science at 'Dr. Madaus & Co.,'" *Social History of Medicine* 14 (2001): 459–82; Eberhard Wolff, "Medizinkritik der Impfgegner im Spannungsfeld zwischen Lebenswelt und Wissenschaftsorientierung," in *Medizinkritische Bewegungen im Deutschen Reich (ca. 1870–ca. 1933)*, ed. Martin Dinges (Stuttgart: Franz Steiner Verlag, 1996), 79–108. The literature on "alternatives" is, in fact, vast, extending far beyond *Naturheilkunde* to include things like mesmerism and popular piety. For a very impressive review of some of this literature, see Michael Saler, "Modernity and Enchantment: A Historiographic Review," in the *American Historical Review* 111 (2006): 692–716.

15. This seems to be true even for college students taking German history courses in the United States, England, and Ireland. A review of H-Net's excellent database of German History syllabi, for example, suggests that German civil society in the Wilhelmine period receives, at best, cursory treatment. This might help to explain why it is still common for students of German history to believe in the myth of an authoritarian, homogenous, and highly interventionist Wilhelmine state. On this point, see Dennis Sweeney, "Reconsidering the Modernity Paradigm: Reform Movements, the Social and the State in Wilhelmine Germany," *Social History* 31 (2006): 405–34.

16. This is an insight borrowed, in part, from the work done by subaltern studies scholars, not least Chakrabarty and Prakash, op. cit. For a few important contributions, see Janet Abu-Lughod, *Before European Hegemony: The World System, AD 1250–1350* (New York: Oxford University Press, 1989); Arjun Appadurai, *Modernity at Large: Cultural Dimensions of Globalization* (Minneapolis: University of Minnesota Press, 1996); Ulrich Beck, *Risk Society: Towards a New Modernity* (London: Sage, 1999); Dipesh Chakrabarty, *Provincializing Europe: Postcolonial Thought and*

Historical Difference (Princeton: Princeton University Press, 2000); Gyan Prakash, *Another Reason: Science and the Imagination of Modern India* (Princeton: Princeton University Press, 1999); Immanuel Wallerstein, *European Universalism: The Rhetoric of Power* (New York: New Press, 2006).

17. Walt Rostow, *The Stages of Economic Development: A Non-Communist Manifesto* (Cambridge: Cambridge University Press, 1960); Samuel Huntington, "The Change to Change: Modernization, Development and Politics," *Comparative Politics* 1971(3): 283–322.

18. For a couple of the key works in this tradition, see Helmut Plessner's *Die verspätete Nation: über die politische Verführbarkeit bürgerlichen Geistes* (Stuttgart: W. Kohlhammer, 1959); Ralf Dahrendorf's *Society and Democracy in Germany* (Garden City, NJ: Doubleday, 1967); Hans-Ulrich Wehler's *Das Deutsche Kaiserreich 1871– 1918* (Göttingen: Vandenhoeck und Ruprecht, 1973).

19. The literature is both voluminous and well known. A recent collection by Helmut Walser Smith, *The Continuities of German History: Nation, Religion, and Race Across the Long 19th Century* (Cambridge: Cambridge University Press, 2008), suggests that a second rethinking is in the works. See also the very productive exchange in *Sehepunkt* 9 (2009), numbers 1 and 9.

20. Historians Michael Geyer and Konrad Jarausch, for example, claim that "the modernization perspective is gradually joining the national narrative and its Marxist alternative as yet another discredited meta-narrative of German history." Michael Geyer and Konrad Jarausch, *Shattered Past: Reconstructing German Histories* (Princeton: Princeton University Press, 2003), 101. Thomas Rohkrämer's work is a good example of this more plural approach. See, for example, *Eine andere Moderne*, op. cit.

21. Hau, 113. More recently, Uwe Heyll ignores the evidence and, indeed, much of what he himself writes, to conclude that classical *Naturheilkunde* was essentially a distillation of petit bourgeois, romantic-era ideology. In this view, simplicity may have simply been a mask for ignorance.

22. This brings us full circle, though, to the problem with modernization theory in the first place: *Progress toward what end?* Peter Dear, *The Intelligibility of Nature: How Science Makes Sense of the World* (Chicago: University of Chicago Press, 2006).

23. It is not my intention to rehash the debate about "social construction." I do, however, think that historians of science have shown us that "science" is as shaped by social, cultural, political, and economic forces as are other areas of human endeavor. The following are just a few of the works (historical and otherwise) that make this case. Thomas Gieryn, *Cultural Boundaries of Science: Credibility on the Line* (Chicago: University of Chicago Press, 1999); Arne Hessenbruch, "Science as Public Sphere: X-Rays Between Spiritualism and Physics," in *Wissenschaft und Öffentlichkeit in Berlin, 1870–1930*, ed. Constantin Goschlar (Stuttgart: Franz Steiner Verlag, 2000), 89–126; Bruno Latour, *Pandora's Hope: Essays on the Reality of Science Studies* (Cambridge, MA: Harvard University Press, 1999). In particular, see chapter 2: "Circulating Reference: Sampling the Soil in the Amazon Forest." Steve Shapin, *A Social History of Truth: Civility and Science in Seventeenth Century England* (Chicago: University

of Chicago Press, 1994); Jan Goldstein, *The Post-Revolutionary Self: Politics and Psyche in France* (Cambridge, MA: Harvard University Press, 2005); Bruno Latour, *The Pasteurization of France*, trans. Alan Sheridan and John Law (Cambridge, MA: Harvard University Press, 1988); Peter Galison and Bruce Hevly, *Big Science: The Growth of Large-Scale Research* (Stanford: Stanford University Press, 1992); Bruno Latour and Steve Woolgar, *Laboratory Life: The Social Construction of Scientific Facts* (Beverly Hills: Sage, 1979); Roger Cooter and Stephen Pumfrey, "Separate Spheres and Public Places: Reflections on the History of Science Popularization and Science in Popular Culture," cited in *History of Science* 22 (1994): 237–67; Robert Johnston, ed., *The Politics of Healing: Histories of Alternative Medicine in North America* (New York: Routledge, 2004); James Whorton, *Nature Cures. The History of Alternative Medicine in America* (Oxford: Oxford University Press, 2002); Corinna Treitel, *A Science for the Soul: Occultism and the Genesis of the German Modern* (Baltimore: Johns Hopkins University Press, 2004).

24. This is essentially the point developed by Susan Pedersen in her "Anti-Condescensionism. Review of *Bodily Matters: The Anti-Vaccination Movement in England, 1853–1907*, by Nadja Durbach," *London Review of Books*, September 1, 2005: 1–9.

25. The public health apparatus in Germany—due in part to the influence of health and hygiene reformers like those at the German League—offers some indication. In Germany, medical doctors, many of them with specialized training in natural therapies, are typically more focused on a holistic approach to health that takes into account patient history, prophylaxis, and environmental concerns than are their Anglo-American counterparts. Lynn Payer, *Medicine and Culture. Varieties of Treatment in the United States, England, West Germany, and France* (New York: Henry Holt and Co., 1988).

26. On the stakes of these different bodily economies, see Durbach, 4–12.

27. As Steve Shapin tells us, the creation of a class of scientific experts makes "[a] more docile public," in part because individuals are less responsible for their own personal well-being. Steve Shapin, "Science and the Public" in *Companion to the History of Modern Science*, R. C. Olby, G. N. Castor et al., eds. (London: Routledge, 1996): 900–1006. I am in no way denigrating the work done by the WHO, or the medical experts who dedicate themselves to saving lives. I only want to suggest that this, too, has unintended consequences.

28. The Institute of Medicine of the National Academies, *The Smallpox Vaccination Program. Public Health in an Age of Terrorism* (sic) (Washington: National Academies Press, 2001), 18.

29. I address these issues in my final chapter.

30. Jürgen Helfricht, *Vincenz Prießnitz (1799–1851) und die Rezeption seiner Hydrotherapie bis 1918. Ein Beitrag zur Geschichte der Naturheilbewegung* (Husum: Matthiesen, 2006), 9–10. According to a 1992 study, more than 70 percent of Germans expressed some level of commitment to natural therapies. The same study determined that more than 60 percent of German doctors had some form of "alternative therapy" as their specialty.

1

1. *Naturheilkunde* did not come into broad usage until at least the 1850s. For this reason, I use "natural therapies" as an umbrella term to describe that complex of diagnostic and therapeutic technologies that would come, in the second half of the nineteenth century, to be known as *Naturheilkunde*. See Karl Eduard Rothschuh, *Naturheilbewegung, Reformbewegung, Alternativbewegung* (Stuttgart: Hippokrates Verlag, 1983).

2. Thomas Lekan and Thomas Zeller, eds., *Germany's Nature: Cultural Landscapes and Environmental History* (New Brunswick, NJ: Rutgers University Press, 2005).

3. John Williams, *Turning to Nature in Germany: Hiking, Nudism, and Conservation, 1900–1940* (Stanford: Stanford University Press, 2007), 3.

4. Uwe Heyll, *Wasser, Fasten, Luft und Licht. Die Geschichte der Naturheilkunde in Deutschland* (Frankfurt: Campus, 2007).

5. Robert Richards, *The Romantic Conception of Life: Science and Philosophy in the Age of Goethe* (Chicago: University of Chicago Press, 2002).

6. Heikki Lempa, *Beyond the Gymnasium. Educating the Middle-Class Bodies in Classical Germany* (New York: Lexington Books, 2007).

7. In the 1980s and 1990s, it became common to talk about "social construction" of all sorts of different things, from ideas and persons, to diseases, animals, the environment, and nature. While the topics and titles are extraordinarily diverse, works on this subject typically share the belief that the world is produced, experienced, and interpreted through an eminently social lens. We create categories in the world, and then those categories act recursively to organize our own ideas and experiences. This was a productive line of inquiry, and it generated some very important work. More recently, though, historians have shown that "social construction" does not adequately account for the phenomenal quality of the world we live in. Death, for example, may be a social reality experienced by the community and mediated in ritual and religious text. Death is *also*, of course, a biological reality that occurs independent of its social construction. Without denying the social and cultural elements of practices and ideas, historians have worked to create a more dynamic way of thinking about them. As environmental historians in particular have shown, the world is not just a script written by human actors. For an excellent collection that examines the interaction between humans and other historical agents (including the built environment, animals, technology, and climate), see Dorothee Brantz, ed., *Beastly Natures: Animals, Humans, and the Study of History* (Charlottesville: University of Virginia Press, 2010). Brantz is influenced by actor-network theory, pioneered by, among others, Bruno Latour. See Bruno Latour, *Reassembling the Social: An Introduction to Actor-Network-Theory* (New York: Oxford University Press, 2005).

8. I explore the period between 1890 and 1918 in chapter 2.

9. This is a point made, in a rather different way, by Ulrich Linse. Linse argues that cultural critics and so-called "nature apostles," while fairly limited in their contemporary significance, served as "incubators" for ideas that would only gain traction years later. Ulrich Linse, 1983.

10. See, for example, Paul Weindling's excellent *Health, Race and German Politics Between National Unification and Nazism, 1870–1945* (Cambridge: Cambridge University Press, 1989).

11. Wilhelm Siegert, "Zur Geschichte der Naturheilbewegung," in *25 Jahre im Dienste der Volksgesundheit. Festschrift zum 25 jährigen Bestehen des Deutschen Bundes der Vereine für naturgemäße Lebens- und Heilweise* (Berlin: Eigener Verlag, 1914), 7–19. Franz von Bielau, *Authentische Biographie von Schlesiens berühmten Naturarzt und Erfinder der Wasserheilkunde* (Freiwaldau: Verlag von Betty Titze, 1902). Robert Jütte, *Geschichte der alternativen Medizin: von der Volksmedizin zu den unkonventionellen Therapien von Heute* (Munich: C. H. Beck, 1996), 116; Janet Browne, "Spas and Sensibilities: Darwin at Malvern," in *The Medical History of Waters and Spas*, ed. Roy Porter (London: Wellcome Institute for the History of Medicine, 1990), 102–13. Here, 102–4. Jane B. Donegan, "*Hydropathic Highway to Health.*" *Women and Water-Cure in Antebellum America* (Westport: Greenwood Press, 1986), 5–6. Philo vom Walde, *Vincenz Prießnitz: Sein Leben und Sein Wirken. Zur Gedenkfeier seines Hundertsten Geburtstages dargestellt* (Berlin: Verlag von Wilhelm Möller, 1899). Passim. Recently, Jürgen Helfricht has used newly discovered archival materials to produce an extraordinary contribution to the study of Prießnitz. Helfricht, 2006.

12. See Christian Andree's introduction to Ernst von Held-Ritt's *Prißnitz* (sic.) *auf Gräfenberg oder treue Darstellung seines Heilverfahrens mit kaltem Wasser* (Würzburg: Bergstadtverlag Wilhelm Gottlieb Korn, 1988—first printed 1837). See, in particular 9 and 14–15.

13. Whether because of his limited education or for other reasons, Prießnitz never produced a body of literature detailing his ideas about health and healing. The various accounts I use to understand water therapies and "nature" cosmologies in the first decades of the nineteenth century are therefore drawn from patients, guests, observers, acolytes, and critics. Vom Walde, 1. Von Bielau, 6.

14. Here I borrow from the Norman Gevitz edited collection *Other Healers: Unorthodox Medicine in America* (Baltimore: Johns Hopkins University Press, 1988).

15. Anon. "Zur Agitation gegen den Kurpfuscherei-Gesetzentwurf," in *Gesundheitslehrer. Volkstümliche Monatsschrift. Offizielles Organ der Deutschen Gesellschaft zur Bekämpfung des Kurpfuschertums* [GL hereinafter] 13 (1910): 120–22. See also Dr. Heinrich Kantor, "Die Wirkung der Prießnitzschen Umschläge," GL 15 (1912): 45. And Dr. Marcus, "Medizin, Naturheilmethode und Kurpfuscherei Part III," a lecture held for the "Liberal Bürgerverein in Hirschberg zu Schlesien" on February 21, 1907. In *Hygienische Blätter. Offizielles Organ der deutschen Gesellschaft zur Bekämpfung des Kurpfuschertums* [HB hereinafter] 3 (1906/07): 53–61.

16. See, as an example, Dr. Wilhelm Winsch, *Wie ich Naturarzt wurde! ein ärztliches Glaubensbekenntnis nach einem im Bürgersaal des Berliner Rathauses gehaltenen Vortrag: mit einem Nachwort über die drohende Aufhebung der Kurierfreiheit* (Berlin: Verlag Lebenskunst-Heilkunst, 1910).

17. This story is likely apocryphal, but for present purposes, this hardly matters. More important is what this kind of story tells us about the different ways that people "saw" and "used" various "nature" concepts.

18. As with much of the Prießnitz story, the details vary. Andree suggests that two surgeons were consulted, while von Bielau notes only one full doctor (*Arzt*). Von Bielau also suggests that there were internal contusions and swelling but does not elaborate. Andree, 11; von Bielau, 11.

19. See, for example, vom Walde, 2–3. Also, von Bielau, 8–11. This story, or variations on this theme, can be found in a variety of published sources. Common to the different iterations of this story is their emphasis on Prießnitz's ability to observe the natural world and translate its laws for human purposes. One thoughtful admirer of Prießnitz did express skepticism over this account. Franz von Bielau suggested that, given the interest in miraculous cures, Prießnitz was likely exposed to stories about notable illnesses and recoveries in the course of evening meals and local gossip. The basic principles of water therapies probably reached him through such interactions. Von Bielau, 10. See also Andree, 10. This point is also made in a review of one Prießnitz biography. See "*Vincenz Priessnitz, sein Leben und Wirken. Zur Gedenkfeier seines hundertsten Geburtstages.* Dargestellt von Thilo (sic.) vom Walde," in *Zeitschrift fur diätetische und physikalische Therapie* [*ZDPT* hereinafter] 4 (1900): 246–48. The history of water cures in Silesia is a long one, but the tradition of storytelling is, after all, even longer. This perfectly reasonable explanation, though, obscures the most illuminating part of the story: in Prießnitz's medical universe, natural laws governed health and illness, and the attentive eye—not necessarily the learned one—could read these laws. This medical universe lived long after Prießnitz had died. This point has also been suggestively developed by Uwe Heyll.

20. Dr. med. Eduard Schnitzlein, cited in vom Walde, 210.

21. Andree, 14. vom Walde, 162–64.

22. The following is based largely on Andree's account. See, in particular, 19–21. Helfricht's work on Prießnitz offers a substantial account. Helfricht, 124ff. See also Vladimir Krizek's very interesting *Kulturgeschichte des Heilbades* (Leipzig: W. Kohlhammer, 1990).

23. Dr. Eduard Oertel, *Oertel-Bauer Lexikon der Naturheilkunde* (Köln: Lingen Verlag, 1962) 62nd edition. First published 1908.

24. Andree, 19–21.

25. Andree, 13. Helfricht offers somewhat lower figures. Helfricht, 151.

26. Helfricht, 111. Vom Walde offers a far higher number, claiming that Prießnitz's income for 1839 alone was 120,000 Gulden. Vom Walde, 31.

27. See, for example, "The Founder of the Cold-Water Cure," *Boston Medical and Surgical Journal* 27 (November 30, 1842): 283. Cited in Donegan, 15, note 14. See also James Wilson and James Manby Gully, *The Dangers of the Water Cure and its Efficacy compared with those of the Drug Treatment of Disease . . . with an account of cases treated at Malvern* (London, 1843); J. Manby Gully, *The Water Cure and Chronic Disease* (London, 1846). Gully and Wilson directed the famous Malvern Hydro, at which such Victorian luminaries as Charles Darwin and Alfred Lord Tennyson were introduced to the "Gräfenberg" cure of Vincenz Prießnitz. For a wonderful discussion of Darwin family at the waters see Browne, 102–13.

28. Von Bielau, 20.

29. Ibid.

30. Ibid., 28.

31. Cited in Donegan, 6.

32. Von Bielau, 19.

33. Dr. Carl Munde, *Memoiren eines Wasserarztes* Volume I (Dresden & Leipzig: in der Arnoldschen Buchhandlung, 1847), 2nd edition. All citations, unless otherwise indicated, are from Volume I. Here, 104. See also vom Walde, 38.

34. Jules Michelet, *Das Meer*, trans. Friedrich Spielhagen (Leipzig: J.J. Weber, 1861). Cited in vom Walde, 230. Vom Walde abbreviates the text. For the full passage, Michelet, 250–51.

35. Munde, 136–37.

36. Heikki Lempa, "The Spa: Emotional Economy and Social Classes in Nineteenth-Century Pyrmont," *Central European History* 35 (2002): 37–73. See also Douglas Mackaman, *Leisure Settings: Bourgeois Culture, Medicine, and the Spa in Modern France* (Chicago: University of Chicago Press, 1998).

37. Lempa (2002), 50–51.

38. They generally agreed, for example, about Prießnitz's extraordinary competence as a healer, and about his contributions to the medical field. This view was shared by advocates of lay healing as well as their critics, though the conclusions they drew were hugely different. They also agreed that a rigorous schedule, relative seclusion from distractions offered by cities and by day-to-day living, and that time in natural settings—as well as exposure to fresh air, clean water, and ample sunlight—were good for healthy bodies, and great for sick ones.

39. Christian Wilhelm Hufeland, *Art of Prolonging Life*, trans. Edmund Wilson (Boston: Ticknor Reed, and Fields, 1854). Based on the 1796 German edition. Heikki Lempa offers a far more subtle reading of this than I can offer here. See Lempa (2007), 27–37.

40. Howard L. Kaye, review of *The Normal and the Pathological*, by Georges Canguilhem, *Journal of Interdisciplinary History* 21 (1990): 141–43. Here, 142.

41. Vom Walde, 66. Italics in the original.

42. Jütte, 30. Trained as a forester, Rausse took seriously Rousseau's imperative to "get back to nature," traveling to North America in the mid-1830s to study the habits of indigenous peoples. During his travels, he contracted typhus and was forced to return to Central Europe. After months of suffering, Rausse went to Gräfenberg in search of a cure. He stayed with Prießnitz for most of 1837 and 1838, first as a patient, and later as an apprentice and helper.

43. J. H. Rausse, *Anleitung zur Ausübung der Wasser-oder Naturheilkunde für Jedermann, der zu Lesen Versteht* (Leipzig: Gesundheitsblätter Verlag, 1895), 4th ed., Book 1, 14.

44. J. H. Rausse, *Anleitung*, Book 2, 71.

45. Rausse, *Anleitung*, Book 3, 7.

46. Natural healers recognized that the healing process did not always work and that the symptoms could sometimes be fatal.

47. Rausse, *Anleitung*, Book 2, 16. Book 3, 7.

48. Hufeland, 300–301.

49. Rausse, *Anleitung*, Book 2, 24–5.

50. Ibid., Book 2, 19.

51. Ibid., Book 2, 20.

52. The causes are too diverse to cite here. The failed 1848 Revolution led to a crackdown on civic associations thought to have potentially political objectives, religious reformers were trying to reconcile Christian belief with the natural sciences, new technologies excited public interest, and explorers were achieving celebrity status. For more on this subject, see also note 76.

53. Weindling, 230 ff. For a fascinating look at the founder of Odol and the driving force behind the Dresden Hygiene Exhibition, Karl August Lingner, see Helmut Obst's *Karl August Lingner. Ein Volkswohltäter?: Kulturhistorische Studie anhand der Lingner-Bombastus-Prozesse 1906–1911* (Göttingen: V & R, 2005).

54. Christine Brecht, "Das Publikum belehren—Wissenschaft zelebrieren. Baketerien in der Ausstellung 'Volkskrankheiten und ihre Bekämpfung' von 1903," 53–76, in Christoph Gradmann and Thomas Schlich, eds., *Strategien der Kausalität: Konzepte der Krankheitsverursachung im 19. und 20. Jahrhundert* (Pfaffenweiler: Centaurus-Verlagsgesellschaft, 1999). Here, 54.

55. Arne Hessenbruch, "Science as Public Sphere: X-Rays Between Spiritualism and Physics," 89–126, in Constantin Goschlar, ed., *Wissenschaft und Öffentlichkeit in Berlin, 1870–1930* (Stuttgart: Franz Steiner Verlag, 2000). Here, 121.

56. Andreas Daum, *Wissenschaftspopularisierung im 19 Jahrhundert: Bürgerliche Kultur, Naturwissenschaftliche Bildung und die deutsche Öffentlichkeit, 1848–1914* (Munich: R. Oldenbourg Verlag, 1998), 27.

57. A variety of articles in *Gesundheitslehrer. Volkstümliche Monatsschrift. Offizielles Organ der Deutschen Gesellschaft zur Bekämpfung des Kurpfuschertums* illuminate this point. See, for example, the short articles "Wo gehen wir heuer hin?" by Dr. Josef Schuster, 63–65; "Die Luftbäder in der Schwindsuchtsbehandlung," anon., 68, and "Erfolglose Badekuren," anon., 70. In *GL* (4)1908.

58. Rausse, *Anleitung*, Book 2, 1.

59. Ibid., Book 2, 72–73, 103. Historian Lester King summarizes the position of John Wesley regarding the medical estate as follows: "Physicians came to be regarded as something more than human and thus had a vested interest in trying to keep at a distance the generality of mankind who might pry into professional mysteries. Highly technical terms came into being, quite unintelligible to the common man." Lester S. King, *The Medical World of the Eighteenth Century* (Chicago: University of Chicago Press, 1958), 36.

60. Rausse, *Anleitung*, Book 2, 12.

61. Vom Walde, 80–83. Ernst von Held-Ritt, 78. The American situation seems to have been, if anything, more extreme. James Whorton, for example, tells of the use of Cayenne pepper in cold-water enemas. James C. Whorton, *Nature Cures. The History of Alternative Medicine in America* (Oxford: Oxford University Press, 2002), 33.

62. Munde, vol. 1, 150.

63. Ibid., 151.

64. In fact, his healing wounds became the object of curiosity and speculation, with one of his particular friends, the Baron Ch——t, suggesting that they analyze the pus resulting from his many boils, a suggestion that Munde politely declined. Ibid., 153.

65. Ibid., 156.

66. Lorenz Gleich, *Nur Kein Wasser! Beiträge zur Begründung der Wasserheillehre in einer Sammlung von Aufsätzen von Dr. Gleich, Wasserarzt in München*, ed. B. Vanoni (Augsburg: Verlag von Lampart und Comp, 1847).

67. Theodor Hahn, *Der Vegetarismus, seine wissenschaftliche Begründung und seine Bedeutung für das leibliche, geistige und sittliche Wohl des Einzelnen, wie der gesammten Menschheit. Ein Beitrag zur Lösung der socialen Frage* (Berlin: Theobald Grieben, 1869); Dr. Med. H. Hennemann, *Das Sündenregister der Medicinheilkunde* (St. Gallen: Verlag von Altweg-Weber zu Kreuzberg, 1875), 2nd edition, 172–181; J. H. Rausse (H. Francke), *Anleitung,* 11–12; Alfred von Seefeld, *Studien über Gesundheit und Krankheit* (Berlin: Theobald Grieben, 1869), 48; Gustav Simons, *Die Überwindung des Kapitalismus. Eine Vorbedingung für die Volksgesundheit* (Oranienburg bei Berlin: Verlag des Deutschen Kulturbundes für Politik, 1913); Gustav Simon, *Das Gesamtbild deutscher Erneurungsbestrebungen. Ein Leitfaden für alle Reformer, besonders für die Führer* (Oranienburg: Wilhelm Möller, 1913).

68. Dr. Lorenz Gleich, *Ueber die Nothwendigkeit einer Reform der Sogenannten Hydrotherapie, oder Geist und Bedeutung der Schrothlichen Heilweise. Nebst einem kurzen Reisebericht als Einleitung* (Munich: Johann Deschler, 1851); Lorenz Gleich, (1847).

69. Lorenz Gleich (1847), 5. For Gleich's definition of this healing force— which borrows heavily from Hufeland—see 67.

70. Dr. Lorenz Gleich, 1851. Interestingly, Gleich also spent time at the Gräfenberg Sanatorium. According to Steinbacher (1862), he was under Prießnitz's care for three months. Jörg Melzer, *Vollwerternährung: Diätetik, Naturheilkunde, Nationalsozialismus, sozialer Anspruch* (Stuttgart: Franz Steiner Verlag, 2003), 69.

71. Gleich (1847), 7–9.

72. K.E. Rothschuh, "Die Konzeptualisierung der Naturheilkunde im 19. Jahrhundert," in *Gesnerus* (1/2) 1981: 175–90. Here, in particular 185–87.

73. Gleich (1851), 18.

74. Lorenz Gleich, *Dr. Gleichs Physiatrische Schriften*, 15, cited in Rothschuh, 186.

75. Gleich (1847), IX.

76. Ibid., 38.

77. Philipp Sarasin, *Reizbare Maschinen. Eine Geschichte des Körpers, 1765–1914* (Frankfurt am Main: Suhrkamp, 2001), 42.

78. Vom Walde, 90–91. After Rausse's death in 1848, Hahn edited and published his mentor's work, a fact that helped to establish his reputation in natural healing circles and to ensure the continued circulation of Rausse's ideas.

79. Vom Walde, 91.

80. Jütte, 155. See also Krabbe, 54–55. Struve allegedly became vegetarian after reading Rousseau's *Emile* in 1832.

81. Advocates for vegetarianism were also concerned with the ethical implications, as evidenced by the extraordinary quote from Seefeld. "Und doch, wenn wir einsehen, daß es nicht der Wille des Schöpfers war, daß wir andere Geschöpfe verzehren sollten, so kommen wir bald dahin, das Schlachten als eine unberechtigte Grausamkeit anzusehen. Und jede andere Grausamkeit, die unter irgend welchem Deckmantel gegen Thiere verübt wird, empört uns umso tiefer als Sie nachwiesbar auch stets zur Grausamkeit gegen Menschen führt." Seefeld, 14. Krabbe, 59. See also Christoph Conti, *Abschied vom Bürgertum: Alternative Bewegungen in Deutschland von 1890 bis heute* (Reinbek bei Hamburg: Rowohlt Verlag, 1984), 68. Seefeld, for example, cited the salutary benefits of dancing and laughing, strolling and good company. Seefeld, 49.

82. This was, after all, a common way of arguing for much of the nineteenth century, one displaced only slowly by clinical and laboratory research in physiology and comparative anatomy. Theodor Hahn (1870), 78, 1st edition 1865. Seefeld makes a similar point, claiming that "der Mensch ist nach seiner ganzen Natur auf Früchte angewiesen, auf Getreide, Obst, Kartoffeln und andere mehrige oder saftige Pflanzentheile." Seefeld, 2–3.

83. Theodor Hahn (1870), 64 ff. He claimed, for example, that "stimulants … are the slayers of instinct." Hahn (1870), 83.

84. The reactionary possibilities here are no doubt obvious. In terms of access to resources, living wages, housing reform, and preventive health care, the progressive possibilities are perhaps less clear, but equally pronounced. Both Hahn and Seefeld, for example, pointed to the issue of sustainability in making the case for vegetarianism. Hahn claimed that vegetables, fruits, nuts, and potatoes were a better use of arable land than were meat products. Hahn (1870), 97. For a similar argument, see Seefeld, 48.

85. Jütte, 155. Steve Shapin has pointed to just such a role for vegetarianism in Britain: while vegetarian societies, because of their numerous proscriptions, were never able to attract members in numbers that other reform societies did, they did function as conceptual pivot points that brought together a variety of reform traditions—religious, ethical, hygienic, body cultural—representing millions and touching the lives of millions more. Steve Shapin, "Vegetable Love: The History of Vegetarianism," *New Yorker,* January 22, 2007.

86. Hahn (1870), 1. Dr. med. Strunckmann claimed that in Germany, confessional freedom had been secure since Luther and that this freedom extended as much to medical matters as it did to religious ones. Dr. med. Strunckmann, "Naturheilbewegung und verwandte Bestrebungen," in *Allgemeiner Beobachter* 1 (1911/12): 17–20. Here, 18.

87. Eduard Baltzer, *Ideen zur Socialen Reform. Sendschreiben an die Hochgeehrte Mexicanische Societät fur Geographie und Statistik in Mexico* (Nordhausen: Verlag Ferd. Fürstemann, 1873), 13, 33.

88. Hahn (1869), III

89. It is at first surprising when one finds nature becoming a category of analysis in religious and social reform contexts, in movements aimed at transforming the clothes

that were worn and the apartments that were built. But this is precisely what happened in German-speaking lands after roughly 1850. One of the keys to the broad circulation of this complex of nature concepts was the emerging relationship between natural healers and religious reformers after roughly the mid-century. Religious reform societies used a language of rational "nature" to make their own case for a less hierarchical, more liberal state church even before the Frankfurt Parliament. Beginning in the early 1840s, Protestant Reform societies like the Free Religious Community claimed that the natural sciences offered the chance to ground ethical values and spiritual longings on an essentially rational footing. Whether as consumers of popular scientific literature, or as nodes in a network that brought young natural scientists and scientific popularizers together with religious and social reformers, the Free Religious Community created the opportunity for seemingly strange alliances to emerge. One such alliance was the relationship between Theodor Hahn and Eduard Baltzer (1814–1887)—a delegate to the 1848 Frankfurt Parliament, the first president of the Free Religious collective (Daum, 208), founder of the first vegetarian association in Germany in 1867–68, and editor of the *Vereinsblatt für Freunde der Naturgemäße Lebensweise* (Barlösius, 45). Daum, 194–96. See also Brederlow, in particular, 50–70.

Natural healers had a clear professional interest in this developing relationship, and it made sense for them to borrow the rhetoric of a reform theology—a rhetoric that would have been broadly familiar to a variety of audiences—in making their case for parity between mainstream medicine and natural alternatives. H. Hennemann, for example, argued that just as the church in Germany had, in the course of the nineteenth century, been turned into a quasi-state institution, so too had medicine come under the aegis of the state, benefiting from all the protections and advantages the state was able to offer. Hennemann (1875), IX. This kind of claim could easily be multiplied.

This language of confessional tolerance became even more useful after 1869, when medicine became one of the free professions, open to citizens regardless of age, religion, or accreditation. Despite these formal guarantees, nonlicensed healers in the tradition of Prießnitz, Rausse, Gleich, and Hahn still faced barriers to entry, and licensed doctors still enjoyed unofficial protections from the state.

90. Daum, 208.

91. Janos Frecot, Johann Friedrich Geist, and Diethart Kerbs, *Fidus, 1868–1948: zur ästhetischen Praxis Bürgerlicher Fluchtbewegung* (Munich: Rogner & Bernhard, 1972), 33; Barlösius, 45.

92. Eduard Baltzer, *Erinnerungen. Bilder aus meinem Leben* (Frankfurt an Main: Verlag des deutschen Vegetarier-Bundes, 1907), 88.

93. Ibid., 68.

94. Ibid.

95. Ibid., 13.

96. Eduard Baltzer, *Vegetarisches Kochbuch für Freunde der natürlichen Lebensweise* (Leipzig: Verlag von H. Hartung und Sohn, 1903), 129, 135; Theodor Hahn, *Makrobiotisches Kochbuch oder: die Kunst, recht zu kochen, gut zu essen, und fröhlich, gesund und lange zu genießen: ein praktisches Handbuch für die Küche des Deutschen*

Volkes (Cothen: Schettler Verlag, 1870); Theodor Hahn, *Kleines Kochbuch für Freunde der naturgemäßen Diät (Vegetarier)* (Köthen: Schettler, 1883); Brederlow, 21. 97. In the years when Prießnitz was practicing, for example, one sees medical textbooks that included sections on the therapeutic uses of water. Ludwig Choulant, *Anleitung zu dem Studium der Medicin* (Leipzig: Voß, 1829); Rudolph Wagner, *Grundriß der Encyklopädie und Methodologie der medizinischen Wissenschaften* (Erlangen: J. J. Palm und Ernst Enke, 1838); C. F. Heusinger, *Grundriss der Encyclopädie und Methodologie der Natur- und Heilkunde* (Eisenach: Chr. Fr. Bärecke, 1839). In fact, balneologie continued to be a minor subfield within academic medicine for most of the century; as a result, an autonomous unit dedicated to balneologie and hydrotherapy was created in 1899 at the annual Congress of Natural Scientists in Aachen. Similarly, German medical researchers pursued a range of different avenues in their efforts to combat disease. Particularly when it came to the study of infectious diseases, researchers consistently asked why some individuals and communities were more affected than others. Here, the problems of individual disposition and environmental conditions were clearly on display. I want to thank an anonymous reviewer for suggestions on this point.

2

1. Thomas Lekan and Thomas Zeller, eds., *Germany's Nature: Cultural Landscapes and Environmental History* (New Brunswick: Rutgers University Press, 2005), 3.

2. The German League for Natural Lifestyle and Therapy Associations was originally founded as *Deutscher Bund der Vereine für Gesundheitspflege und arzneilose Heilweise*, but changed its name in 1900 to *Deutscher Bund der Vereine für naturgemäße Lebens- und Heilweise*. I use Michael Hau's translation here. *The Cult of Health and Beauty in Germany: A Social History, 1890–1930* (Chicago: University of Chicago, 2003). Hereafter I refer simply to The German League.

3. Friedrich Eduard Bilz, *Der Zukunftsstaat: Staatseinrichtung im Jahre 2000* (Leipzig: F. E. Bilz, 1904). Socialists, too, were fond of imagining the future. August Bebel, *Zukunftsstaat und Sozialdemokratie* (Berlin: Vorwärts, 1893).

4. "Naturist" is the term used by John Williams to describe people and groups that "attempted to reorient the German people towards nature." John Williams, *Turning to Nature in Germany: Hiking, Nudism, and Conservation, 1900–1940* (Stanford: Stanford University Press, 2007), 2.

5. Klaus Bergmann, *Agrarromantik und Großstadtfeindshaft* (Meisenheim am Glan: Hain, 1970); George Mosse, *The Crisis of German Ideology: Intellectual Origins of the Third Reich* (New York: Schocken Books, 1981); Fritz Stern, *The Politics of Cultural Despair: A Study in the Rise of the Germanic Ideology* (Berkeley: University of California Press, 1961).

6. Pierre Bourdieu, *Distinction: A Social Critique of the Judgement of Taste*, trans. Richard Nice (Cambridge MA: Harvard University Press, 2000).

7. Michael Cowan, *Cult of the Will: Nervousness and German Modernity* (University Park, PA: Pennsylvania State University Press, 2008); Hau, op. cit.

8. Sven Oliver Müller and Cornelius Torp, eds., *Das Deutsche Kaiserreich in*

der Kontroverse (Göttingen: Vandenhoeck & Ruprecht, 2009), 14–16, 20.

9. Some outstanding correctives are Carsten Timmermann's "Rationalizing 'Folk Medicine' in Interwar Germany: Faith, Business, and Science at 'Dr. Madaus & Co.,'" *Social History of Medicine* 14 (2001): 459–82; Williams, op. cit.; Jeffrey K. Wilson, "Environmental Protest in Wilhelmine Berlin: The Campaign to Save the Grünewald," *German Historical Institute Bulletin* 3 (2006): 9–25. See also the excellent review articles by Edward Ross Dickinson, "Not So Scary After All? Reform in Imperial and Weimar Germany," *Central European History* 43 (2010): 149–72; Dennis Sweeney, "Reconsidering the Modernity Paradigm: Reform Movements, the Social and the State in Wilhelmine Germany," *Social History* 31 (2006): 405–34. The case is put most forcefully by Young-Sun Hong, "Neither Singular nor Alternative: Narratives of Modernity and Welfare in Germany, 1870–1945," *Social History* 30 (2005): 133–53.

10. Franz-Josef Brüggemeier, Mark Cioc, and Thomas Zeller, eds., *How Green Were the Nazis? Nature, Environment, and Nation in the Third Reich* (Athens: Ohio University Press, 2005). While the collection determines that the Nazis ultimately impacted "green" movements in a negative way, the provocative framing of the problem does point to the widespread perception of close ties between National Socialism and "naturist" ideas and practices.

11. When the German League was founded in 1889, it had 142 associations with some 19,000 members. Just 25 years later, there were more than 800 associations, between them offering some 10,000 lectures annually, and boasting almost 150,000 dues-paying members. Regin (1995), 49–51. Florentine Fritzen, 176. See Williams, 2007; Wolfgang Krabbe, *Gesellschaftsveränderung durch Lebensreform: Strukturmerkmale einer sozialreformerischen Bewegung im Deutschland der Industrialisierungsperiode* (Göttingen: Vandenhoeck und Ruprecht, 1974). For further discussion of the Life-reform movement, please see my introduction to the book.

12. The German League counted 145,272 members in 1912. Of those 27.7 % identified themselves as industrial workers, with another 35 % identifying themselves as artisans or craftsmen. The explicitly socialist League for People's Health counted just 11,500 members in 1912. For absolute figures, see *Nature's Doctor (Naturarzt) NA* 40 (1912): 1–3. I refer to *Nature's Doctor* as *NA* in subsequent notes. For the demographic breakdown, see Regin (1995), 80. For figures on the League for People's Health, see *Volksgesundheit* [VG hereinafter] 22 (1912): 50–53. HstaL PP-V 1824. *Verein für Volksverständliche Gesundheitspflege Leipzig Süd-Ost (1890–1936)*.

13. As Magnus Hirschfeld put it, "He who submits to nature will be happy and healthy, he who rejects it, sick and wretched. We can only truly enjoy the triumph of culture when we maintain our connection to nature." Magnus Hirschfeld, "Die Hauptgesichtspunkte der Naturheilbewegung," *NA* 26 (1898): 203. In a different vein, Adolf Damaschke captures the attitude of the German League toward political neutrality:

Eins nach außen, Kampfgewaltig,
All um ein Panier geschart,
Doch nach innen vielgestaltig,
Jeder frei nach seiner Art.

Adolf Damaschke, *Die Organisation der deutschen Naturheilbewegung* (Berlin: Verlag von Wilhelm Möller, 1896). For similar sentiments, see *NA* 17, issue 4 (1889); *NA* 17, issue 7 (1889); *NA* 17, no. 12 (1889); *NA* 18, issue 3 (1890).

14. Oskar Mummert, "Welche sozialhygienischen Forderungen ergeben sich aus den Prinzipien der Naturheilkunde?" *NA* 41 (1913): 49. Cited also in Regin (1995), 255.

15. Staatsarchiv Leipzig PP-V 118. *Verein für Gesundheitspflege und arzneilose Heilweise Leipzig Neustadt-Reudnitz* to the district court on November 27, 1907.

16. According to Reinhold Gerling, who edited the *German League's* monthly publication *Nature's Doctor* from 1898–1906, the group's mission was "Health through Enlightenment." Reinhold Gerling, "Neujahr 1898!" *NA* 26 (1898): 1–3.

17. Stadtarchiv Leipzig Kap. 35, Nr. 915. *Association for Natural Healing Leipzig Gohlis* to the Leipzig city council on January 1, 1909. Emphasis in the original.

18. Magnus Hirschfeld, *"Staatshilfe oder Selbsthilfe?"* *NA* 25 (1897): 66. His arguments about "self-help" line up nicely with his advocacy for the decriminalization of homosexuality. Hirschfeld believed that homosexuality was a biological fact not subject to choice and that prosecution of homosexual acts amounted to an attack on nature. He called on authorities to focus their attention instead on sexual predators and "Johns" who did, in his view, have the freedom to make choices. Magnus Hirschfeld, "Ein Programmentwurf für die deutsche Naturheilbewegung, Teil II," *NA* 25 (1897): 167–69.

19. Magnus Hirschfeld, *"Staatshilfe oder Selbsthilfe?"* *NA* 25 (1897): 67.

20. For an excellent treatment of some of these issues, Cornelia Regin, op. cit.

21. A. Knoll, "Eine Aufgabe der Naturheilbewegung," *NA* 26 (1898): 33–36.

22. Tilman Harlander, "Zentralität und Dezentralisierung—Großstadtentwicklung und städtebauliche Leitbilder im 20. Jahrhundert," in Clemens Zimmermann, ed., *Zentralität und Raumgefüge der Großstädte im 20. Jahrhundert* (Stuttgart: Franz Steiner Verlag, 2006), 23–25; Brian Ladd, *Urban Planning and Civic Order in Germany, 1860–1914* (Cambridge, MA: Harvard University Press, 1990), 14; Marianne Rodenstein, *Mehr Licht, mehr Luft: Gesundheitskonzepte im Städtebau seit 1750* (Frankfurt am Main: Campus Verlag, 1988), 115.

23. Hermann Wolf, "Die Gesundheitspflege des Arbeiters (II)," *Neue Heilkunst* 13 (1901): 12. See also S. Milton Rabson, "Alfred Grotjahn, Founder of Social Hygiene," *Bulletin of the New York Academy of Medicine* 12 (1936): 43–58. For an important historical contribution, see Corinna Treitel, "Max Rubner and the Biopolitics of Rational Nutrition," *Central European History* 41 (2008): 1–25.

24. Dr. med. Georg Bonne, *"Über die Notwendigkeit einer systematischen Dezentralisation unserer Großstädte in hygienischer, sozialer und volkswirtschaftlicher Beziehung, II,"* *Monatsschrift für Soziale Medizin* 1 (1904): 373; Beate Witzler, *Großstadt und Hygiene: Kommunale Gesundheitspolitik in der Epoche der Urbanisierung* (Stuttgart: Franz Steiner Verlag, 1995), 92–130.

25. Jeffrey K. Wilson develops this argument in reference to environmental protection in Berlin between roughly 1904 and 1914. Wilson, op. cit.

26. Alexander Knoll, *"Eine Aufgabe der Naturheilbewegung,"* *NA* 26 (1898): 33.

27. Alexander Knoll, "Naturheilbewegung und Koalitionsrecht," *NA* 26 (1898): 316–18.

Alexander Knoll, "Naturheilbewegung und Lebensmittelzölle," *NA* 29 (1901): 208–10.

28. My discussion here collapses important distinctions between social democratic and left-liberal reformist projects. For a subtle analysis of different kinds of reformist agendas in Wilhelmine Germany, see Sweeney, op. cit. in particular, 411–19.

29. Cited in Ingrid Matthäi, "Kleingartenbewegung und Arbeitergesundheit," *Medizin, Gesellschaft und Geschichte* 13 (1994): 193. Members of the Association for Healthcare and Non-Medicinal Healing in Leipzig Reudnitz-Neustadt claimed that parks, gardens, bathing, and sport facilities were all tools to insulate the working poor from the "corrupting effects of street-life." Stadtarchiv Leipzig Kap. 35, Nr. 779. *Verein fur Gesundheitspflege L.-Ost zu Leipzig Reudnitz und Leipzig Neustadt* to the city council on February 6, 1905.

30. For an excellent contribution, see Dennis Sweeney, "Cultural Practice and Utopian Desire in German Social Democracy: Reading Adolf Levenstein's Arbeiterfrage," *Social History* 28 (2003): 174–201.

31. Adolf Levenstein, *Die Arbeiterfrage. Mit besonderer Berücksichtigung der sozialpsychologischen Seite des modernen Grossbetriebes und der psycho-physischen Einwirkungen auf die Arbeiter* (Manchester, NH, 1975), 188. First published 1912.

32. Ibid., 350.

33. Adolf Damaschke, who helped to found the German Land Reform and Garden City movements, helped to forge these linkages. After editing *Nature's Doctor* between 1894 and 1896, he left to pursue the issue of land reform full time. Franz Schönenberger and Oskar Mummert also held long-time advisory positions.

34. Anna Pappritz, "Die Wohnungsfrage," *NA* 37 (1909): 179–83.

35. Bund Deutscher Bodenreformer, *Adolf Damaschke zu seinem 50. Geburtstage* (Franfurt Oder: Trowitzsch, 1915), 12.

36. Rodenstein, op. cit., 107.

37. W. Heinrich, "*Was jeder von der Bodenreform wissen sollte*," *NA* 35 (1907): 281–82.

38. Ibid.

39. For a good overview of these issues, see Justizrat Dr. Liertz, *Adolf Damaschke und die Deutsche Bodenreform* (Düsseldorf: L. Schwann, 1948); Adolf Damaschke, *Die Bodenreform: grundsätzliches und geschichtliches zur Erkenntnis und Überwindung der sozialen Not* (Jena, 1918—15th edition).

40. Wilhelm Siegert, "*Nationalökonomie*," *NA* 38 (1910): 25.

41. Bund Deutscher Bodenreformer, op. cit., 9.

42. Paul Schirrmeister, "Bodenrecht und Volksgesundheit," *NA* 35 (1907): 86–88.

43. Paul Schirrmeister, "Gartenstadt und Volksgesundheit," *NA* 35 (1907): 167–170.

44. Ibid. My emphasis.

45. Clemens Zimmermann and Jürgen Reulecke, eds., *Die Stadt als Moloch,*

Land als Kraftquell? Wahrnehmungen und Wirkungen der Großstädte um 1900 (Basel: Birkhäuser, 1999). A more productive line seems to be the one advanced by Moishe Postone, who argues that the preoccupation with "speculation" is a typical populist misrecognition of the nature of capital, one that reduces complex economic processes to simple explanations. In this context, "fetishized anti-capitalism" has close ties to popular anti-Semitism. I am not convinced, though, that land reform *does* simplify political economy in the way that Postone's analysis suggests. Land reformers were, after all, concerned primarily with issues of urban overcrowding from a public health standpoint. Interestingly, Damaschke made a similar argument in his 1891 pamphlet *Manchestertum, Antisemitismus oder Bodenbesitzreform?* (Berlin: Thormann u. Goetsch, 1891). Damaschke argued that land reform was an important way of blunting the appeal of popular anti-Semitism. While I am not convinced by the argument, Postone's work represents a line of inquiry deserving of further historical study. Moishe Postone, "History and Helplessness: Mass Mobilization and Contemporary Forms of Anticapitalism," *Public Culture* 18 (2006): 93–110. I want to thank David Spreen for suggesting this point.

46. Paul Schirrmeister, "Gartenstadt und Volksgesundheit," *NA* 35 (1907): 167–70.

47. Dickinson, op. cit., 170–72.

48. Damaschke, 1896; Regin, op. cit., 250.

49. Ulla Terlinden and Susanna von Oertzen, *Die Wohnungsfrage ist Frauensache! Frauenbewegung und Wohnreform 1870–1933* (Berlin: Reimer, 2006); *NA*, passim.

50. Schönenberger, op. cit., IV.

51. Joachim Joe Scholz, "*Haben wir die Jugend, so haben wir die Zukunft.*" *Die Obstbausiedlung Eden/Oranienburg als alternatives Gesellschafts- und Erziehungsmodell (1896–1936)* (Berlin: Weidler, 2002), 36; Regin, op. cit. 249–50.

52. H. Krecke, "Eine Bodenreform-Kolonie in Deutschland. Die vegetarische Obstbaukolonie Eden bei Oranienburg," *Deutsche Volksstimme* 9 (1898): 4–12; Otto Jackisch, "Die Obstbaukolonie Eden, ihre Gründung, Wachsen und jetziger Zustand," *Deutsche Volksstimme* 14 (1903): 432–37; Anonymous, *Die Obstbausiedlung Eden in Oranienburg in den ersten 25 Jahren ihres Bestehens* (Oranienburg: Eden, 1920).

53. For a far more comprehensive discussion of the Wilhelmine reform milieu, see Kevin Repp, *Reformers, Critics, and the Paths of German Modernity: Anti-Politics and the Search for Alternatives* (Cambridge, MA: Harvard University Press, 2000).

54. Bilz, op. cit., 1071; Reinhard Spree, *Soziale Ungleichheit vor Krankheit und Tod: zur Sozialgeschichte des Gesundheitsbereichs im Deutschen Kaiserreich* (Göttingen: Vandenhoeck & Ruprecht, 1981).

55. Bilz, op. cit., 1071.

56. Reinhold Gerling was well known to contemporaries in Wilhelmine reform circles and achieved sufficient notoriety to find himself cited in the pages of the *Deutsche biographische Enzyklopädie, Geistige Berlin,* in countless newspaper stories, and in almost as many legal proceedings. According to one biographer, Gerling

published some 4,000 articles and 118 books about various reform causes, from sex education and hypnotism, to antivivisection and the occult. Walter Gerling, *Reinhold Gerling. Sein Leben und Wirken. Biographische Skizze mit 3 Abbildungen* (Oranienburg: Orania Verlag, 1923), 25; Helmut Obst, *Karl August Lingner. Ein Volkswohltäter? Kulturhistorische Studie anhand der Lingner-Bombastus Prozesse, 1906–1911* (Göttingen: V & R Unipress, 2005), 94; Richard Wrede und Hans von Reinfels, *Das Geistige Berlin: eine Enzyklopädie des geistigen Lebens Berlins* Bd. 1 (Berlin: Verlag von Hugo Storm, 1897), 132. Gerling has also started to crop up in the Anglophone historical literature. See, for example, Michael Cowan's *Cult of the Will: Nervousness and German Modernity* (University Park: Pennsylvania State University Press, 2008).

57. Schönenberger, cited in Mummert, "25 Jahre Naturarzt," 105.

58. StdtL, Kap. 35, Nr. 396. *Geschäftsbericht des Vereins für naturgemäße Gesundheitspflege—Leipzig Kleinzschocher, 1894–1914.*

59. StdtL. Kap. 35, Nr. 1807. *Naturheilverein zur Möckern- -Wahren. 1896–1940.* Broschüre: *Naturheilverein Möckern.*

60. StaL PP-V 1824. Akten betr. den *Verein für Volksverständliche Gesundheitspflege Leipzig Süd-Ost. Flugblatt des Naturheilvereins Leipzig-Ost. "Was Wollen die Naturheilvereine?"* Article 2.

61. The association *Wasserfreunde*, for example, planned to build a "worthy temple" on Kommandantenstraße in central Berlin. *Landesarchiv Berlin* 232 01 Nr. 1 Bd. 1.

62. Wilson, op. cit., 17–18. Wilson analyzes the campaign to protect the Grünewald, which lasted from roughly 1904 to 1914. Efforts to protect green space in and around Berlin were already picking up steam around the turn of the century. See, for example, Julius Matern, "An den Magistrat zu Charlottenburg," *Deutsche Volksstimme* 12 (1901): 42–44; Adolf Damaschke, "Wie Stehts um Dahlem"? *Deutsche Volksstimme* 12 (1901): 193–95.

63. T. C. Horsfall, *The Improvement of the Dwellings and Surroundings of the People. The Example of Germany* (Manchester: University Press, 1904), 25.

64. The *Reichstag* even voted for a tax on unearned capital gains as a measure to control land speculation. The tax was in place from 1911–1913. Ladd, op. cit., 196. For one of the more famous contemporary pieces, see Rudolph Elberstadt, *Handbuch des Wohnungswesens und der Wohnungsfrage* (Jena: Gustav Fischer, 1909).

65. Wilhelm Siegert, "Wohnungsnot," NA 40 (1912): 168.

66. Williams, op. cit., 2–3.

67. *Bäder Album der Königlich Preußischen Domänen Verwaltung* (Aachen: Aachener Verlag u. Druckerei Gesellschaft, 1900), 8.

68. Warren Maurer, *Understanding Gerhardt Hauptmann* (Columbia: University of South Carolina Press, 1992), 142; Thomas Mann, *The Magic Mountain: A Novel*, trans. John E. Woods (New York: Knopf, 1995); Joachim Radkau, *Max Weber: die Leidenschaft des Denkens* (Munich: Hanser, 2005); Peter Thomas, "Being Max Weber," *New Left Review* 41 (2006); Edith Hanke, "Max Weber, Leo Tolstoy and the Mountain of Truth" in Sam Whimster, ed., *Max Weber and the Culture of Anarchy* (New York: St. Martins, 1999): 144–61.

69. Hannes Siegrist, Hartmut Kaelble, and Jürgen Kocka, eds., *Europäische*

Konsumgeschichte: zur Gesellschafts- und Kulturgeschichte des Konsums (18. bis 20. Jahrhundert) (Frankfurt: Campus, 1997); Alon Confino and Rudy Koshar, "Regimes of Consumer Culture: New Narratives in Twentieth-Century German History," *German History* 19 (2001): 135–61.

70. Eberhard Wolff, "Kultivierte Natürlichkeit: zum Naturbegriff der Naturheilbewegung," *Jahrbuch des Instituts für Geschichte der Medizin der Robert Bosch Stiftung* 6 (1986): 219–36.

71. Williams *op. cit.* In particular, the introduction and chapter 1.

72. Adolf Just, *Return to Nature*, trans. H. A. Nisbett (London: G. Routledge & Sons, 1912), 49.

73. For a contemporary review of some of the medical literature, see "Bücherbesprechung," *Therapeutische Monatshefte* 22 (1908): 484–86.

74. Dr. Georg Liebe, "Luft- und Sonnenbäder in Heilstätten für Lungenkranke," *Zeitschrift für physikalisch-diätetische Therapie* (subsequently *ZpdT*) 11 (1908): 197–204.

75. Humboldt *Universitätsarchiv—Medizinische Fakultät* 1386, Fiche 3–4. Medical Faculty to Konrad Haenisch in reference to the creation of a chair for *Naturheilkunde*, 1919.

76. Sander Gilman, *Franz Kafka* (London: Reaktion, 2005), 68.

77. For an early treatment of clothing reform and body culture, see Krabbe, 1974, 93–112.

78. Albert Shaw, "The Therapeutic Value of the Air-Bath," *American Monthly Review of Reviews* 35 (1907): 632. My emphasis.

79. William Paul Gerhard, *Modern Baths and Bath Houses* (Boston: Stanhope Press, 1908), 219.

80. Wolff, *op. cit.*, 221.

81. Arnold Rikli, *Die Grundlehre der Naturheilkunde einschließlich die atmosphärische Cur* (Leipzig: L. Fernau Verlag, 1895), 22–23. " . . . den civilisierten Menschen . . . mit der Atmosphäre vertraut zu machen." I have taken some liberty with this translation, using "outdoors" in place of "Atmosphäre." Ultimately, I feel that this captures the sense of the passage more clearly.

82. *Stadtarchiv Leipzig.* Kap. 35, Nr. 383. *Verein fur Naturheilkunde Leipzig-West.* Association report to the city council on May 3, 1916.

83. *Stadtarchiv Leipzig.* Kap. 35, Nr. 779. *Verein fur Gesundheitspflege L.-Ost zu Leipzig Reudnitz und Leipzig Neustadt.* Association report to the city council on March 29, 1905.

84. *Geheimes Staatsarchiv Preußischer Kulturbesitz* (Subsequently GStaPK) I HA Rep 77. Title 719, Nr. 26, Beiheft 1 (II), 9935.

85. Ibid. The emphasis was in the ministry copy.

86. Ibid. Nor was it only the women from the Women's Association for the Advancement of Morality (DFVHS) who were scandalized. A local worker reported that, while repairing the roof of an adjacent property, he observed the pastor himself taking the sun in the nude. He made no mention of the naked women.

87. GStaPK I HA Rep 77. Title 719, Nr. 26, Beiheft 1 (II), 12064, Berlin,

October 7, 1899.

88. GStaPK I HA Rep 77. Title 719, Nr. 26, Beiheft 1 (IIA), 1716.

89. Ibid. Title 719, Nr. 26, Beiheft 1 Abschrift I.C 9201.

90. Ibid. Title 719, Nr. 26, Beiheft 1 9935.

91. Ibid.

92. John Fout makes a parallel argument about homosexuality. See his "Sexual Politics in Wilhelmine Germany: The Male Gender Crisis, Moral Purity, and Homophobia" in John Fout, ed., *Forbidden History: The State, Society, and the Regulation of Sexuality in Modern Europe* (Chicago: University of Chicago Press, 1992).

93. Regin, op. cit.

94. Ibid., 49–51.

95. Reinhold Gerling, "Ruckblick und Ausblick," *NA* 29 (1901): 1–2.

96. Anon., "Erklärung," *Blätter für Volksaufklärung (Neue Heilkunst)* 20 (1908): 18. In January 1909, for example, Gerling cancelled a lecture because there were "only" 212 people in the audience. "Unsere Agitation," *Blätter für Volksaufklärung (Neue Heilkunst)* 21 (1909): 19.

97. Kai Buchholz et al.

98. Cited in Krabbe, op. cit., 13.

99. Christoph Conti, *Abschied vom Bürgertum: Alternative Bewegungen in Deutschland von 1890 bis Heute* (Reinbeik bei Hamburg: Rowohlt, 1984); Green, op. cit.; Ulrich Linse, 1983; Elisabetta Borone, Matthias Riedl, and Alexandra Tischel, eds., *Pioniere, Poeten, Professoren. Eranos und der Monte Verità in der Zivilisationsgeschichte des 20. Jahrhunderts* (Würzburg: Königshausen & Neumann, 2004).

100. Fritzen, 176.

101. F. E. Bilz, *Das Neue Naturheilverfahren: Lehr und Nachschlagebuch der naturgemäßen Heilweise und Gesundheitspflege* (Leipzig: F. E. Bilz, 1898).

102. Fritzen, op. cit., 47–48.

103. Ibid.

104. Julian Marcuse, *Bäder und Badewesen in Vergangenheit und Gegenwart. Eine Kulturhistorische Studie* (Stuttgart: Enke Verlag, 1903). Philipp Sarasin has shown how this preoccupation with daily practice was closely related to a new concern with hygiene and medical prevention. Philipp Sarasin, *Reizbare Maschinen. Eine Geschichte des Körpers, 1765–1914* (Frankfurt am Main: Suhrkamp, 2001).

105. Hong, op. cit.

106. This is what Dirlik meant when he proposed "thinking of the future in terms of alternative historical trajectories that defy the colonization of the future by current structures of power." Arif Dirlik, *The Postcolonial Aura: Third World Criticism in the Age of Global Capitalism* (Boulder, CO: Westview, 1998), 17.

3

1. Geoffrey Cocks and Konrad Jarausch, eds., *German Professions, 1800–1950* (New York: Oxford University Press, 1990).

2. There was a brief interlude during the Jacobin phase of the revolution in

which medicine in France was similarly freed of questions of accreditation. This period began with the law of March 2, 1791, which abolished all trade associations and guilds, and persisted until 1803. See Maurice Crosland, "The *Officiers de Santé* of the French Revolution: A Case Study in the Changing Language of Medicine," *Medical History* 48 (2004): 229–44.

3. Claudia Huerkamp, *Der Aufstieg der Ärzte im 19. Jahrhundert. Vom gelehrten Stand zum Professionellen Experten. Das Beispiel Preußens* (Göttingen: Vandenhoeck & Ruprecht, 1985), 242.

4. Ibid., 255.

5. Ibid.

6. Mary Lindemann, *Health and Healing in Eighteenth Century Germany* (Baltimore: Johns Hopkins University Press, 1996); Lester King, *The Medical World of the Eighteenth Century* (Chicago: University of Chicago Press, 1958); W. F. Bynum and Roy Porter, eds., *Medical Fringe and Medical Orthodoxy, 1750–1850* (London: Croom Helm, 1987). For an outstanding collection that deals with the American example, see Norman Gevitz, ed., *Other Healers: Unorthodox Medicine in America* (Baltimore: Johns Hopkins University Press, 1988).

7. Even in 1880, just 25 % of medical associations canvassed in a national survey expressed strong concerns about the activities of nonlicensed healers. Huerkamp, 259.

8. Here I borrow from the title of Norman Gevitz's edited volume. Gevitz, op. cit.

9. In 1897, for example, doctors concerned about the spread of "quackery" founded a monthly journal designed to educate medical doctors and the interested public about the dangers of sham healers, and by November 1900, major medical associations were forming commissions that would devote themselves exclusively to the "problem" of nonlicensed practitioners. Hsta PK IHA Rep 76 VIIIB, # 1328. The Medical Association for Berlin-Brandenburg to the executive ministerial advisor for the Ministry of Ecclesiastical, Educational, and Medical Affairs, November 14, 1900. In 1900, doctors also founded a professional defense organization informally called the *Leipzig League*. The *Leipzig League* played a key role in bringing all university-trained doctors under the aegis of one professional organization, using a variety of coercive measures to do so.

10. Hsta PK IHA Rep 76 VIIIB, # 1330. Holz cited in *"Zur Bekämpfung des Sogenannten Kurpfuscherei."* June 4, 1903. *Deutsche Tageszeitung.*

11. Hsta PK IHA Rep 76 VIIIB (1328). *"Sammlung auf M3658/97 betr. Ausscheidung der Ärzte aus der Gewerbeordnung. Zusammenstellung der auf den Erlaß vom 9. Oktober, 1897 eingegangenen Berichte der Regierungs- und Oberpräsidenten betr. die infolge der Kurierfreiheit auf gesundheitlichen Gebieten gegenwärtig herrschenden Zustände."*

12. Ibid.

13. Dr. Carl Alexander, "Das Kurpfuschertum und seine Gegner," *GL* 13 (1910): 258–61. Here, 258.

14. Anon., *"Eine Erklärung des Reichsamtes des Innern über die Zahl der Kurpfu-*

scher," *GL* 17 (1914): 28. See also the figures cited for Berlin in 1897 above.

15. Hsta PK IHA Rep 76 VIIIB, # 1329. Leipzig, October 23, 1900.

16. Hsta PK IHA Rep 76 VIIIB, # 1329. "Bekanntmachung, betreffend öffentliche Anzeigen von Heilmitteln und Heilmethoden," published in *Deutsche Medizinische Wochenschrift,* June 5, 1902.

17. Hsta PK IHA Rep 76 VIIIB, # 1329. *Kölnische Zeitung* July 11, 1902.

18. Hsta PK IHA Rep 76 VIIIB, # 1329. Minister of Ecclesiastical Affairs to the Chancellor, August 22, 1902.

19. Hsta PK IHA 76 VIIIB, # 1328. The Ministry of Ecclesiastical Affairs to the Minister of the Interior and the Minister of Trade and Industry, November 14, 1901.

20. Hedwig Herold-Schmidt, "Ärztliche Interessenvertretung im Kaiserreich 1871–1914," in Robert Jütte, ed., *Geschichte der deutschen Ärzteschaft* (Köln: Deutscher Ärzte-Verlag, 1997): 65–66.

21. Even foreign observers noted the way that health and lifestyle entrepreneurs used the media to "sweep away the hard-earned savings of the credulous middle and lower classes." In the same piece, the *British Medical Journal* referred dismissively to the "'Prophet' Bilz." Anon., "Natural Healers in Germany," *British Medical Journal* 2517 (1909): 801.

22. Herold-Schmidt, 50.

23. Ibid., 93.

24. Hsta PK IHA Rep 76 VIIIB, # 1330. *"Die Aufhebung der Kurierfreiheit."* September 19, 1903. *Deutsche Warte.* The text was highlighted in the archival copy, presumably in the Ministry of Ecclesiastical Affairs.

25. Hsta Pk I HA Rep 77, Tit. 719, # 26. Minister of Ecclesiastical Affairs to District Governors and Police Chiefs, June 28, 1902.

26. Hsta PK IHA Rep 76 VIIIB, # 1330. *"Verein für Gesundheitspflege und Naturheilkunde* (Freiberg) to the Prussian Ministry for Culture," September 30, 1903. The same petition can be found in the *Hauptstaatsarchiv* in Dresden. HstaD III.III.III, # 15232. *"Verein für Gesundheitspflege und Naturheilkunde* (Freiberg) to the [Saxon] State Minister of the Interior Metzsch." September 22, 1903.

27. Hsta PK IHA Rep 76 VIIIB, # 1327. *Denkschrift betreffend die Aufhebung der Kurierfreiheit und das Verbot der Kurpfuscherei.* From the association of practicing natural healers to the Ministry for Ecclesiastical Affairs. Undated though probably presented in 1896 or 1897.

28. Hsta PK IHA Rep 76 VIIIB, # 1330. *"Verein für Gesundheitspflege und Naturheilkunde* (Freiberg) to the Prussian Ministry for Culture [sic]" September 30, 1903.

29. Hsta PK IHA Rep 76 VIIIB, # 1329. *Kölnische Zeitung,* July 11, 1902.

30. Ibid.

31. Hsta PK IHA Rep 76 VIIIB, # 1329. Chief of Police von Windheim to the Minister of Ecclesiastical Affairs, July 12, 1902.

32. Ibid.

33. Hsta PK IHA Rep 76 VIII B, # 1329. Graf von Schwerin to the Provin-

cial Governor.

34. Hsta PK IHA Rep 76 VIIIB, # 1329. Minister of Ecclesiastical Affairs to the Provincial Governors, December 31, 1902.

35. Hsta PK IHA Rep 76 VIIIB, # 1331. *Über die am 12 Dezember 1904 im Reichsamte des Innern gepflogenen komissarischen Verhandlungen über die Grundzüge eines Gesetzes, betr. die Bekämpfung der Kurpfuscherei.*

36. Hsta PK IHA Rep 76, VIIIB, # 1331. *Abschrift, der Reichskanzler,* January 21, 1908.

37. *Der Kampf um die Augen-Diagnose. Stenographischer Bericht des Felke-Prozesses vor dem Landgericht Crefeld vom 27 Oktober bis 3. November 1909* (Crefeld: Verlag von Albert Fürst Nacht, 1909), 156.

38. Ibid., 14.

39. The loam cure employed healing clay that acted as a kind of plaster, limiting movement and soothing tender regions.

40. Ibid.

41. *Der Kampf,* 176–77. See also the arguments developed by Dr. Kröner, 92.

42. Dr. Emil Schlegel, *Die Augendiagnose des Dr. Ignaz von Peczély* (Tübingen, Verlag von Franz Fues, 1906), 5.

43. *Der Kampf.* Felke, 8.

44. Ibid., 9.

45. Ibid.

46. Ibid. Bellachini, 18–19.

47. Ibid., 63–64.

48. Ibid. Neustätter, 51–52.

49. While it is not entirely clear what was meant here, Bouillon was used in the preparation of the dyptheria vaccination. Felke may have been referring to a vaccination-related illness. "How Antitoxine is made. Report of Consul General Mason of Frankfort [sic], Germany," *New York Times,* January 20, 1895: 28.

50. *Der Kampf.* Neustätter, 52.

51. Ibid.

52. Ibid., 159.

53. Ibid. Dr. Spohr, 34.

54. Ibid. Dr. Ziegelroth, 35.

55. Ibid., 176–77. See also the arguments developed by Dr. Kröner on this line, 92.

56. Ibid. Schulze, 162.

57. Ibid., 166.

58. Ibid., 169. This point of view was not confined just to defenders of lay healing. Rudolf Virchow made a similar point in 1902 when he asked, "Where are the boundaries between quackery and real science? All too often, legislation, court decisions, the activities of the police, *but also, let us not forget, scientific judgement,* are confounded by this problem." BA R/1501. Nr. 109130. Bd. 1. *Acta Betreffend: die Maßregeln zur Bekämpfung der Kurpfuschertums.* June, 1899 to February, 1904. Rudolf Virchow, *Auszug aus "Zum neuen Jahrhundert."* Erschienen in Heft I, Bd. 159—

Seite 3–6—*Archiv fur Anatomie und Physiologie* (June, 1902).
59. Ibid. Klein, 120.
60. *GL* 9 (1909): 173–74.
61. Hsta PK IHA Rep 76 VIIIB, # 1332. *Auszug aus den Verhandlungen des Reichstags.* 90th Session, 1910, 3278–3308. Dr. Delbrück.
62. Ibid.
63. Ibid. Dr. Fassbender.
64. Ibid.
65. Ibid. Emphasis added.
66. Ibid. Zietsch.
67. Ibid.
68. Ibid. Emphasis added.
69. Ibid.
70. Ibid.
71. Ibid.
72. Ibid.
73. Ibid. Dr. med. Arning.
74. Ibid.
75. Hsta PK IHA Rep 76, # 1332. *"Auszug aus den Verhandlungen des Reichstags.* 91st Session, 1910: 3009–3325. Dr. Mayer.
76. Ibid.
77. Ibid.
78. Ibid. The *DSP* was part of the *Wirtschaftliche Vereinigung.* Lattmann is known, in part, for his outspoken anti-Semitism.
79. BA R/8034II, # 1808. *"Das Kurpfuschereigesetz im Reichstage,"* Deutsche *Tageszeitung,* December 1, 1910.
80. BA R/8034II, # 1808. *"Protestversammlung gegen den Entwurf des Kurpfuschereigesetzes,"* Berliner Tageblatt, December 8, 1910.
81. Ibid.
82. Hsta PK IHA Rep 76 VIIIB, # 1329. *"Die Bekämpfung der Kurpfuscherei,"* Nationale Zeitung, July 11, 1902.
83. BA R/1501, # 109135. *Beschlüsse der 20. Kommission zu dem Entwurf eine Gesetzes gegen Mißstände im Heilgewerbe.*
84. Hsta PK IHA Rep 76 VIIIB, # 1329. Berliner Tageblatt, *"Ein Versuch mit unzureichenden Mittlen,"* July 11, 1902. See also Berliner Tageblatt, *"Presse und Kurpfuscherei,"* July 29, 1902.
85. Cornelie Usborne, *Cultures of Abortion in Weimar Germany* (New York: Berghahn Books, 2007), 94.
86. Hill Gates, "The Commoditization of Chinese Women," *Signs* 14 (1989): 799–832.
87. Victor Turner, *The Forest of Symbols: Aspects of Ndembu Ritual* (Ithaca: Cornell University Press, 1967).
88. HstaD III.III.III # 15232. *Abschrift aus dem Jahresbericht des Bezirksarztes*

zu Bautzen auf das Jahre 1904. Dr. Streit, Bezirksarzt.

89. Ibid.

90. Ibid.

91. HstaD III.III.III # 15232. State Medical Council to the Ministry of the Interior in response to Streit's above-cited report on possible connections between natural healers and miscarriages, February 8, 1906.

92. Ibid.

93. Ibid.

94. Usborne, 101.

95. Hsta PK IHA Rep 76 VIIIB, # 1332. *Auszug aus den Verhandlungen des Reichstags.* 90th Session, 1910, 3278–3308. Dr. Delbrück.

96. Unlike his predecessor, Bernhard von Bülow, Bethmann-Hollweg was committed to a policy of centralizing power in the hands of bureaucratic and administrative elites. One socialist critic described him as a "routinizer of governmental praxis *(Routinier der Regierungs-praxis)."* Max Maurenbrecher, "Bethmann-Hollweg," *Sozialistische Monatsheft* Vol. 1(1910): 120.

97. Rolf Neuhaus, *Arbeitskämpfe, Ärztestreiks, Sozialreformer. Sozialpolitische Konfliktregelung 1900–1914* (Duncker & Humblot: Berlin, 1986), 274ff.

98. Huerkamp, 290.

99. According to Neuhaus, the *Leipzig League* participated in 1090 negotiations between 1900–1912. Of these, they won concessions in 984 cases (98%). Negotiations failed in 21 cases, and 85 conflicts were not resolved. Neuhaus (1986), cited in Herold-Schmidt, 93.

100. Huerkamp, 285–96.

101. Ibid., 291.

102. Ibid., 80.

103. Julian Fräßdorf, *Auszug aus den Verhandlungen des Reichstags.* 153rd Session 1905, 4924.

104. Cited in Fräßdorf, 4925.

105. Herold-Schmidt, 85.

106. Ibid.

107. Anon., "Cölner Ärztestreik," *NA* 37 (1909): 134. First reported in the *"Rheinische Zeitung."*

108. BA R/8034II, # 1807. *"Die Ärzte gegen Bethmann-Hollweg,"* Berliner Tageblatt, February 19, 1909.

109. BA R/8034II, # 1807. *"Verärgerte Terroristen,"* Leipziger Volkszeitung, March 6, 1909.

110. Bethmann-Hollweg, cited in ibid.

111. Ibid.

112. HstaD III.III.III. Saxon State Medical Council to the Ministry of the Interior, November 12, 1911. Italics are mine.

113. Anon., *"Zur Jahreswende,"* NA 40 (1912): 1–3. Here, 1. 114. Anon., *"Die Vergewaltigung der Naturheilbewegung während des Krieges,"* NA 47 (1919): 22–25.

Here, 23.

    115. Ibid.

    116. Regin, 445.

4

    1. See chapter 3 for a full discussion of these issues.

    2. Mary Lindemann, *Health and Healing in Eighteenth Century Germany* (Baltimore: Johns Hopkins University Press, 1996); Lester King, *The Medical World of the Eighteenth Century* (Chicago: University of Chicago Press, 1958); W. F. Bynum and Roy Porter, eds., *Medical Fringe and Medical Orthodoxy, 1750–1850* (London: Croom Helm, 1987).

    3. Hermann Canitz, "Ursachen und Wirkungen," *NA* 1 (1889): 6–9. Here, 7.

    4. This kind of view was actually fairly widespread, and in fact, we saw it in the last chapter in comments made by Martin Fassbender in parliament. Canitz's comments prefigured those of Fassbender by more than two decades. Another good example, written at about the time that Fassbender made his comments, can be seen in Hans Freimark, "Das Problem des Kurpfuschertums," *Allgemeiner Beobachter. Halbmonatsschrift für alle Fragen des modernen Lebens* (AB) 1 (1911): 116–19.

    5. Canitz, 7.

    6. Ibid., 8.

    7. *ApdT*, 10 (6), 1908. Dr. med. Krone, "Wissenschaftliche und unwissenschaftliche Therapie," 168–69. Here, 169. The criticism of medical dogma was widespread, as we saw in both the Felke trial and parliamentary hearings in the last chapter. Krone, himself a medical doctor, warned that medicine could not behave as if it were the "papal church."

    8. Wilhelm Siegert, "*Die Sachverständigen im Prozess Canitz in der Beleuchtung der Medizinheilkunde*," Report of the *Berliner Zeitung* cited in *NA* 1 (1889): 204–206. Here, 204.

    9. This was, for example, the view expressed by one petitioner writing to demand the closure of a school for *Naturheilkunde* in Berlin. HstaPK, IHA rep. 76 VIIIB, # 1330. Dr. Med. Hugo Davidsohn to the Minister of Ecclesiastical Affairs, June 24, 1903.

    10. Steve Shapin, in *A Social History of Truth: Civility and Science in 17th Century England* (Chicago: University of Chicago Press, 1994). See, for example XXVI, 6, 25, and 414–15. Thomas Gieryn also offers key insights into the way that person, place, and power serve to shape the way that "science" is known. See for example X–XII, 1–3, and 19 in his *Cultural Boundaries of Science. Credibility on the Line* (Chicago: University of Chicago Press, 1999).

    11. Carsten Timmermann's excellent essay on some of these themes helped to shape the present chapter. See Carsten Timmermann, "Rationalizing 'Folk Medicine' in Interwar Germany: Faith, Business, and Science at 'Dr. Madaus & Co.,'" *Social History of Medicine* 14 (2001): 459–82.

    12. Roger Cooter points out that historians tend to reinforce the belief that

science is "culturally transcendent and bereft of ideological contents," and suggests that this kind of belief reinforces an essentially whiggish understanding of scientific progress. Roger Cooter and Stephen Pumfrey, "Separate Spheres and Public Places: Reflections on the History of Science Popularization and Science in Popular Culture." Cited in *History of Science* 22 (1994): 237–67. This view has largely fallen out of the history and sociology of medicine, and from medical anthropology. For a great introduction to some different approaches to these issues, see Deborah Lupton's *Medicine as Culture. Illness, Disease, and the Body in Western Societies* (London: Sage, 2003).

13. Thomas Schlich and Ulrich Tröhler, eds., *The Risks of Medical Innovation: Risk Perception and Assessment in Historical Context* (London: Routledge, 2006).

14. In an unusually dramatic essay, Dr. Dobrick claimed that the only group that the public despised more than doctors was psychiatrists. Unfortunately for Dobrick, he was a psychiatrist. See his essay "Odium Psychiatricum," *Psychiatrisch-Neurologischen Wochenschrift* 13 (1911): 381–83.

15. Regin, 38.

16. See Carsten Timmermann's *Weimar Medical Culture: Doctors, Healers and the Crisis of Medicine in Interwar Germany, 1918–1933* (Diss: University of Manchester, 1999).

17. Dr. Leyden and Dr. Goldscheider, "Vorrede." In *Zeitschrift für diätetische und physikalische Therapie* 1 (1), 1898: 5–9. Here, 5. Krone, 169; Regin, 38–39.

18. Emil Kraepelin. *100 Years of Psychiatry*, trans. Wade Baskins (New York: Philosophical Library, Inc., 1962), 117. This was, in fact, a fairly common usage, as we shall see below. Kraepelin's text was originally published in 1918.

19. This demographic fact had important consequences for the growing field of social hygiene and the emerging one of racial hygiene. Paul Weindling, *Health, Race and German Politics Between National Unification and Nazism, 1870–1945* (New York: Cambridge University Press, 1989), 15, 17, 33.

20. D. von Engelhardt, "Kausalität und Konditionalität in der modernen Medizin," in *Pathogenese: Grundzüge und Perspektiven einer Theoretischen Pathologie*, ed. H. Schipperges (Berlin: Springer Verlag, 1985), 32–58. Here in particular 32–34.

21. Dr. Ziegelroth, "Was wir wollen," in *Archiv für physikalisch-diätetische Therapie in der ärztlichen Praxis. Offizielles Organ des Ärzte-Vereins für physikalisch-diätetische Therapie* [*ApdT* hereinafter] 1 (1899): 1–3. Here, 1.

22. Ibid.

23. Ernst von Leyden and Alfred Goldscheider, "Vorrede," in *Zeitschrift fur diätetische und physikalische Therapie*. 1 (1898): 5–9. Here, 6.

24. Ibid., 7.

25. Another instance that points to the growing acceptance of physical and dietary therapies was the creation of an autonomous section for balneology and hydrotherapy at the 1899 Congress of Natural Scientists in Aachen. Dr. Julian Marcuse, "Berichte über die Naturforscherkongress in Aachen," *ZdpT* 4 (1900): 534–36.

26. W. A. Securius, "An die Mitglieder des Bundes der Vereine für naturgemäße Lebens und Heilweise," *Neue Heilkunst* [*NH* hereinafter] 12 (1900): 73.

27. Anon., *NH* 12 (1900): 170.

28. See, for example, Anon., "Die Naturheilbewegung," *Hygienische Blätter* 1(1904): 7–12. Here, 10.

29. Dr. W. E. "Ein Vorschlag zum Frieden," reprinted from the *Physiatrische Rundschau, NA* 33 (1905): 153–56.

30. See notes 22 and 24 above.

31. Dr. W. E., 155.

32. Ibid.

33. Ibid., 156.

34. The creation of *ApdT and ZdpT* is one broad indicator of this trend. Heyll tells us that, by 1902/3, 142 doctors were employed as association doctors for local natural healing associations. Heyll, 2006, 174.

35. Dr. med. Kleinschrod, "Ein Vorschlag zum Frieden: Erwiderung von Dr. Kleinschrod," *NA* 33 (1905): 182–84.

36. Ibid., 182.

37. Reinhold Gerling, "Der Weg zum Frieden," *NA* 34 (1906): 281–83. Here Gerling responded to an article of the same name published in the *Neue Stader Zeitung* by Dr. Bachmann.

38. Dr. Bachmann, cited in Gerling, *NA* 34 (1905): 281–82.

39. Ibid., 282.

40. Ibid.

41. On this point, see once again Gieryn. See also Carsten Timmermann, 2001.

42. Reinhold Gerling, "Anerkennung," *NA* 25 (1897): 97–98.

43. Ibid.

44. An Association of Practitioners of *Naturheilkunde* was founded in 1891 with an eye to formalizing the training of prospective natural healers. This association had 294 members in 1907. Heyll (2006), 151.

45. The resolution was brought on May 25, 1919. Dr. Beyer (SPD), Dr. Hermann Weyl (USPD), Emil Abderhalden (DDP), Dr. Faßbender (Zentrum), and Dr. Schloßmann (Zentrum).

46. R. C. Hentschel, *Franz Schönenberger, 1865–1933. Biobibliographie eines ärztlichen Vertreters der Naturheilkunde* (Med. Diss. Munich: Ludwig-Maximilians Universität, 1979), 121–22. Alfred Brauchle, *Zur Geschichte der Physiotherapie. Naturheilkunde in ärztlichen Lebensbildern* (Heidelberg: Haug Verlag, 1971), 149. The archival record suggests that Dr. Weyl may have played a key role in drafting the Ausschuß, if only because his is the only version of the draft legislation to be preserved in the archive. *HUA. Med. Fak.* 1386, Fiche 7, April 11, 1919.

47. *HUA Med. Fak.* 1386, Fiche 7. Undated circular.

48. *HUA Med. Fak.* 1386, Fiche 3–4. Undated circular.

49. Hentschel, 123. Goldscheider was, of course, one of the founding editors of *ZdpT*.

50. Ibid., 136.

51. Petra Werner, "Zu den Auseinandersetzungen um die Institutionalisierung von Naturheilkunde und Homöopathie an der Friedrich-Wilhelms Universität

zu Berlin zwischen 1919 und 1933," *Medizin, Gesellschaft und Geschichte* 13 (1993): 205–19. Here, 210. In at least one instance, this included collaboration with right-extremist student groups hostile not just to the social democratic administrators intervening in university politics, but also to the Jewish candidates that were sometimes nominated. Daniel Jung, *Institutionalisierung und akademische Ausbildung auf dem Gebiet der Naturheilkunde im gesellschaftlichen Wandel. Die Geschichte der Lehrestühle für Naturheilkunde an den medizininschen Fakultäten Jena (1923–1938) und Berlin (1900–1945)* (Leipzig, Diss: Universität Leipzig, 1995), 18–19.

52. Hentschel, 124.

53. Werner, 209–10.

54. Hentschel, 124.

55. *HUA* Med. Fak. 1386, Fiche 3–4. Medical Faculty to Minster Haenisch in reference to the creation of a chair for *Naturheilkunde*. Undated circular.

56. Ibid., Fiche 3–4. Undated circular.

57. Ibid., Fiche 3–4. Undated circular, 3–4.

58. This is the tack taken by medical men working to scuttle a proposal to build an out-patient clinic for *Naturheilkunde* at a hospital in the Grambke district of Bremen. Wagschal, 1913.

59. *HUA* Med. Fak. 1386, Fiche 3–4. Undated circular, 7.

60. Ibid., Fiche 3–4. Undated circular, 14.

61. In 1905, for example, the University of Berlin made permanent a provisional institute for hydrotherapies that had both clinical and teaching facilities. Interestingly, Kraus failed to mention the example of Ernst Schweninger. Dr. Ernst Schweninger was director of a clinic at the Charité and Bismarck's personal doctor. After Bismarck's death, Schweninger was offered the directorship of the newly opened hospital in Berlin Groß-Lichterfelde. That hospital became the first public facility in Germany to specialize in physical and dietary therapies. Georg Schwarz, *Ernst Schweninger. Bismarcks Leibarzt* (Leipzig: Verlag Philipp Reklam, 1941), 61–62. It is true that, after sustained battles with the Berlin Medical Association, Schweninger gave up his directorship in 1906. *Reformblätter. Illustrierte Zeitschrift für alle hygienischen Reformen und für volksverständliche Gesundheitspflege.* 5 (2), 1902. Anon., "Zum Kampf der Ärzte gegen die Naturheilkunde," 46–47. Nevertheless, the hospital in Berlin Groß-Lichterfelde continued to offer patients the option of treatment using physical and dietary therapies.

62. Klein did eventually find a university position, taking a chair for *Naturheilkunde* at the University of Jena in 1924. Jung, 23.

63. Hentschel, 126.

64. While Schönenberger's nomination was intended as a show of compromise—he was, after all, a medically trained doctor who called for greater collaboration between natural healers and medical men—Haenisch had no real intention of compromising on the broader issue. Whatever objections the medical faculty had, Haenisch was committed to seeing an advocate for natural healing in the open chair. Werner, 209. Haenisch took a similarly unyielding approach in his support for Alfred Grotjahn as full professor for social hygiene at the University of Berlin. See M.

Hubenstorf, "Alfred Grotjahn," in *Berlinische Lebensbilder: Mediziner*, eds. W. Treue and R. Winau (Berlin: Colloquium Verlag, 1987): 337–58. Here, 355; S. M. Rabson, "Alfred Grotjahn, Founder of Social Hygiene," *Bulletin of the New York Academy of Medicine* 12 (1936): 43–58. Here, 53.

65. *HUA* Med. Fak. 1386, Fiche 7, March 22, 1920.

66. Ibid.

67. Schönenberger, 1898.

68. Schönenberger, 1906; 1911.

69. *HUA* Med. Fak. 1386, Fiche 7, March 22, 1920.

70. Ibid.

71. Siegert, 204.

72. *HUA* Med. Fak. 1386, Fiche 7, March 22, 1920.

73. Not only had he been a practicing natural healer *before* he received his medical degree, but *after* receiving his license, he returned immediately to that milieu from which he had come, advocating the prerogative of lay healers as editor of *Nature's Doctor*.

74. Hentschel, 143. Heyll, 183.

75. Hentschel, 128–29.

76. HstaPK, IHA rep. 76 VIIIB, # 1330, Sept. 14, 1903. *Betrifft Antrag des praktischen Arztes Dr. Davidsohn auf eventuelle Schließung der hier bestehenden sogenannten Fachschulen für Naturheilkundigen.*

77. Timmermann (2001), 463.

78. HstaPK, IHA rep. 76 VIIIB, # 1330. Dr. Med. Hugo Davidsohn to the Minister of Ecclesiastical Affairs, June 24, 1903.

79. Reinhold Gerling, "Anerkennung," *NA* 25 (1897): 97–98.

5

1. The WHO statement announced that "'the world and its peoples have won freedom from smallpox, which was a most devastating disease sweeping in epidemic form through many countries since earliest time, leaving death, blindness and disfigurement in its wake and which only a decade ago was rampant in Africa, Asia and South America.'" Cited in Hugh Pennington, "Smallpox and Bioterrorism," *Bulletin of the World Health Organization* 81 no. 10 (2003): 762–67. The success of the global smallpox campaign seemed, on the surface at least, to vindicate targeted interventions, and one consequence of this was the massive expansion of the global pharmaceutical industry. The developing world became a testing ground for new products. Global public health presented vast new market opportunities.

2. In India alone, 152,000 Indian "health workers" were involved in the smallpox eradication campaign. Press release: South Asia Region of the World Health Organization, "WHO commemorates 30 years Freedom from Smallpox," <http://www.searo.who.int/en/Section316/Section503/Section2557_15052.htm>

3. Paul Greenough, "Intimidation, Coercion, and Resistance in the Final

Stages of the South Asian Smallpox Eradication Campaign, 1973–1975," *Social Science and Medicine* 41 no. 5 (1995): 633–45. For an excellent broad-gauged discussion and a helpful bibliography, see Sanjoy Bhattacharya, *Expunging Variola: The Control and Eradication of Smallpox in India, 1947–1977* (New Delhi: Orient & Longman, 2006).

4. Ibid. Even some of those involved in the campaign recognized and commented on the parallels.

5. Vincente Navarro, "A Critique of the Ideological and Political Positions of the Willy Brandt Report and the WHO Alma Ata Decision," *Social Science and Medicine* 18 no. 6 (1984): 467–74. As Navarro notes, WHO interventions have regularly had the effect of de-politicizing large-scale medical interventions. In this context, the spread of infectious disease is dissociated from the broader social, political, and economic contexts in which it occurs.

6. Andreas Daum, *Wissenschaftspopularisierung im 19. Jahrhundert: bürgerliche Kultur, naturwissenschaftliche Bildung und die deutsche Öffentlichkeit, 1848–1914* (Munich: R. Oldenbourg, 1998). For the American example, see Robert Johnston's excellent *The Radical Middle Class: Populist Democracy and the Question of Capitalism in Progressive Era Portland, Oregon* (Princeton: Princeton University Press, 2003).

7. As Nadja Durbach writes for the British case, "Whether or not children could survive a vaccination both immune from smallpox and relatively unscathed, however, is only part of the issue. The procedure was clearly incompatible with many shared cultural attitudes towards disease and its prevention. . . . Throughout the nineteenth and twentieth centuries, compulsory vaccination was at odds with both popular understandings of bodily economy and assumptions about the boundaries of state intervention in personal life." Nadja Durbach, *Bodily Matters: The Anti-Vaccine Movement in England, 1853–1907* (Durham: Duke University Press, 2005), 4. Vaccination is once again the subject of debate. In particular, parents and some doctors have argued that there is a link between MMR vaccination and autism. The topic found its way onto the cover of *Time* magazine, June 2, 2008. "The Truth About Vaccines," by Alice Park.

8. Hervé Bazin, *The Eradication of Smallpox. Edward Jenner and the First and Only Eradication of a Human Infectious Disease*, trans. Andrew Morgan and Glenise Morgan (New York: Academic Press, 2000), plates 1, 10.

9. Professor Dr. Martin Kirchner, *Schutzpockenimpfung und Impfgesetz* (Berlin: Richard Schoeß, 1911), 14. Louis XV died of smallpox in 1774.

10. The Institute of Medicine of the National Academies, *The Smallpox Vaccination Program. Public Health in an Age of Terrorism* (Washington: National Academies Press, 2001), 11–12. See also Bazin, 4. There are, of course, similar and related viruses that affect animals, of which cow pox is one important example.

11. There are two main types of the disease, Variola major and Variola minor. Variola minor typically has more mild symptoms and has a fatality rate of roughly 1%. Variola major has a fatality rate roughly 30 times that of Variola minor. Ibid., 12.

12. The symptoms typically begin to show ten to twelve days after infection. Kirchner, 7.

13. This phase typically begins ten days after the patient has experienced initial symptoms.

14. Kirchner, 7–8.

15. Ibid., 17.

16. Arthur Allen, *Vaccine. The Controversial Story of Medicine's Greatest Lifesaver* (New York: W. W. Norton, 2007), 37. Practices anticipating those pioneered by Jenner were first introduced to Europe by Lady Mary Wortley Montagu, who had her son "variolated" in Constantinople in 1718, according to the custom of the Greeks and Ottoman Turks. Allen suggests that variolation dates back at least a thousand years. Allen, 27.

17. Allen cites a 1901 case in New York in which as many as 90 people died of tetanus after being vaccinated. Allen, 70.

18. And in fact, Jenner was not the first to use this procedure. "As early as 1713, Salger, the author of *De Lue Vaccarum*, had called attention to the protective power of cowpox," while "[p]robably the first person to vaccinate with bovine virus for prophylactic purposes was Benjamin Jesty, a farmer of Downshy . . . who operated on his wife and two children in 1744." Bernhard Stern, *Should We Be Vaccinated? A Survey of the Controversy in its Historical and Scientific Aspects* (New York: Harper & Brothers Publishers, 1927), 5–6. Stern, a sociologist at Columbia University, believed that Yes, we should!

19. *Vaccinia* is simply cow lymph material.

20. Because cow lymph material was often in short supply, it was common to vaccinate one child with cow lymph and then harvest lymph material from a fresh pustule on the patient to inject directly into other children. See, for example, Eberhard Wolff, *Einschneidende Massnahmen. Pockenschutzimpfung und traditionale Gesellschaft im Württemberg des frühen 19. Jahrhunderts,* (Stuttgart: Franz Steiner Verlag, 1998), 134–35.

21. Axel Helmstädter, "Zur Geschichte der deutschen Impfgegnerbewegung," in *Geschichte der Pharmazie,* 42 (1990): 19–23. Here, 20.

22. Wolff (1998).

23. Allen, 53.

24. Contemporary doctors thought of vaccination as evidence of rational participation in the life of the nation. Thus, one contemporary likened the introduction of vaccination to the introduction of a translated gospel. And he argued that the poor and the uneducated would set themselves against this innovation in the same way they had to the book of common prayer. Wolff (1998), 26.

25. Andreas Holger Maehle, "Präventivmedizin als wissenschaftliches und gesellschaftliches Problem: Der Streit über das Reichsimpfgesetz von 1874," in *Medizin, Gesellschaft und Geschichte,* 9 (1990): 127–48. Helmstädter; Wolff (1998).

26. See Stern (1927), 118, 128, and 131, for example.

27. For the range of these arguments, see Bazin, particularly 128–33. Some thought that anti-vaccine activists were simply contrarian. A British example is instructive. Blanchard Jerrold, a journalist, "critiqued anti-vaccinationists as victims of 'public opinion,' manipulated into fighting for any cause. The anti-vaccination leagues,

he proclaimed in 1883, belonged in the company of '[t]he Association for the Total Suppression of White Hats! The Anti-Flowers in the Button-Hole League! The Society for the Abolition of Green Tea Drinking,''' and so on. Cited in Durbach, 42.

28. Wolff (1996), 85.

29. Dr. C. G. G. Nittinger, *Die Impfung ein Mißbrauch*, (Stuttgart: Emil Ebner, 1867. 1st edition: 1852). Historians have rightly made much of Nittinger's role in shaping anti-vaccine agitation. See, for example, Wolff (1996), 81, and Hemstädter, 20. The caption on the front page of Nittinger's passage read, "Under the German oak sits grieving Germania. At her feet lies her daughter, noble liberty, slain by three vaccine incisions, by which state power takes from every German the freedom to control his own body [*die freie Verfügung über seinen Leib.*] Science must turn away in shame. … The church counts births and deaths, and hides the deficit in its ledgers. On a pox infected cow sits the *Lanzknecht* [*sic*], the modern Don Quixote … with lancet poised to bring the Moloch of vaccination a new victim. … Germany's garden—a field of corpses!" Nittinger, title plate.

30. The Imperial Office of Health, *Blattern und Schutzpockenimpfung. Denkschrift zur Beurtheilung des Nutzens des Impfgesetzes vom 8. April 1874 und zur Würdigung der dagegen gerichteten Angriffe* (Berlin: Julius Springer, 1900), 63.

31. The child's parents would be given an exemption only if they were able to provide a medical certificate stating that vaccination would endanger the child's health, or if they could prove that the child had contracted and survived naturally occurring smallpox.

32. The Imperial Office of Health (1900), 75.

33. For the text of the law, amendments, and discussion, see Dr. O. Rapmund, *Die gesetzlichen Vorschriften über die Schutzpockenimpfung. Reichs-Impfgesetz nebst den dazu gehoerigen Bundesrats-Beschlussen und den in den einzelnen Bundestaaten erlassenen Ausführungsbestimmungen* (Leipzig: Verlag von Georg Thieme, 1900).

34. Paul A. L. Mirus, *Die Impffrage und der Verband deutscher Impfgegner* (Dortmund: Verlag von Robert Keßler, 1910), 5.

35. As Lorraine Daston writes, "The cult of numbers has been the cult of precision since at least the 17th century." Daston reviewing *The History of Statistics: The Measurement of Uncertainty before 1900*, by Stephen Stigler, in *The Journal of Modern History* 61 (1989): 135–37. Here, 135. See also her *Classical Probability in the Age of Enlightenment* (Princeton: Princeton University Press, 1988); Theodore Porter, *Trust in Numbers: The Pursuit of Objectivity in Science and Public Life* (Princeton: Princeton University Press, 1995).

36. Helmstädter, Maehle, Wolff (1996).

37. Maehle and Helmstädter in particular.

38. Arguments about the on-the-ground production of scientific knowledge have been famously made by Bruno Latour in his *Laboratory Life: The Construction of Scientific Facts* (Princeton: Princeton University Press, 1986); Karin Knorr-Cetina, *Epistemic Cultures: How the Sciences Make Knowledge* (Cambridge: Harvard University Press, 1999).

39. Friedrich Bock (Social Democrat) claimed that the medical establishment's power derived from its relationship with the state. *Stenographische Berichte*

über die Verhandlungen des Deutschen Reichstages (SB hereinafter), 243rd Session (28.4.1914): 8291.

40. In an 1873 debate, for example, the left-liberal Dr. Wilhelm Löwe compared smallpox mortality in the civilian population with that of military conscripts. Pointing to far higher incidences of smallpox deaths in the civilian population, Löwe argued that there was a clear correlation between vaccination and the survival of smallpox: while conscripts were vaccinated upon joining military service, and revaccinated after 18 months, the civilian population was only partially vaccinated, and even less frequently revaccinated. For Löwe, these gross data pointed to the real protection vaccination offered, promising increased security through a fully vaccinated population. Faced with intense and unexpected scrutiny, it did not take long for his arguments to fall apart: in the period set aside to evaluate the legislation, a variety of commentators argued that comparing conscript-aged men with the general population skewed results in unacceptable ways. Not only were infants and small children more susceptible to smallpox than were others, but military men had already passed a relatively rigorous physical examination, making them one of the populations least susceptible to infectious disease. Maehle, 130.

41. Ibid., 132.

42. Ibid., 133.

43. Löwe, cited in Heinrich Böing, *Tatsachen zur Pocken- und Impffrage. Eine statistisch-ätiologisch-kritische Studie* (Leipzig: Breitkopf & Härtel, 1882), 42.

44. Böing, VI.

45. Kirchner (1911), 101.

46. Böing, 38.

47. Ibid., 38–39.

48. Ibid., 44.

49. Cited in ibid., 53. Emphasis added.

50. Maehle and Humm are quick to dismiss the use of statistics by critics of compulsory vaccination as "the quantification of their own prejudices." But as Wolff has argued, this is not ultimately the salient point. As he puts it, "Non-specialist critics of vaccination availed themselves of the same kinds of arguments as the experts they criticized." Wolff, 105–6. See also Derrick Baxby, *Smallpox Vaccine, Ahead of Its Time. How the Late Development of Laboratory Methods and Other Vaccines Affected the Acceptance of Smallpox Vaccine* (Berkeley: The Jenner Museum, 2001), 3.

51. H. Hennemann, *Die Impfvergiftung der Jugend des deutschen Reichs.* (1875—no publication data).

52. Eugen Bilfinger, *Ueber fuer und wider den Impfzwang* (Stuttgart: Kommissionsverlag von Konrad Wittwer, 1883). Friedrich Thiele (Social Democrat), SB 153rd Session (27.2.1902). In a 1907 pamphlet, Dr. Karl Strunckmann informed readers at the Ministry of the Interior that, for generations to come, historians would view the early twentieth century as the time when Germans finally "took responsibility for health and healing . . . into their own hands, just as 400 years earlier . . . the laity wrested responsibility for the care of the soul from the Priests." Dr. med. Karl Strunckmann, *Die Naturheilkunde und Ihre Praktischen Vertreter in Gegenwart und Zukunft* (Wolfenbüttel: Verlag von Julius Zwißler, 1907). BA R/1501 Nr. 109134.

Akten Betreffend: die Maßregeln zur Bekämpfung des Kurpfuschertums. Okt. 1909 bis Nov. 1910. Pamphlet delivered to the Ministry of the Interior on November 12, 1909.

53. Imperial Office of Health (1900), 92. In 1877 there were roughly 30,000 signatories, while by 1891, the number had climbed to 90,661.

54. Mirus, 5.

55. See file sets detailing individual cases of alleged vaccine-related illness. Hsta PK IHA VIIIB Kultusministerium Nr. 3990–3994 (*Einzelne Fälle von aufgetretenen Impfschädigungen*).

56. See Dr. Heinrich Oidtmann, *"Dr. H. Oidtman als Impfgegner vor dem Polizeigericht: Weshalb ich meine Kinder nicht habe impfen lassen. Eine Vertheidigungsschrift"* (Duesseldof: Druck von P. Bitter, 1878); Professor Dr. phil. Heinrich Molenaar, *Impftod. Bibliographie der internationalen medizinischen Literatur über Impfschaden, Nutzlosigkeit der Impfung und Verwandtes* (Dortmund: Verlag Robert Kessler, 1912).

57. For a contemporary introduction to the theory and practice of vaccination, see Director of the Berlin Vaccine-Center Dr. M. Schulz, *Impfung, Impfgeschäft und Impftechnik. Ein kurzer Leitfaden für studierende und Ärzte* (Berlin: Richard Schoetz, 1892). Kirchner offers an account two decades later. It is surprising how little had actually changed. Kirchner, 41–43.

58. Peter Frosch, *Bericht über die Thatigkeit der con dem Herrn Minister der Geistlichen Unterrichts und Medizinal Angelegenheiten eingesetzten Kommissin zur Prüfung der Impfstofffrage* (Berlin: Julius Springer, 1896), 58.

59. Martin Kirchner, *Die preussichen Impfanstalten* (Jena: Verlag von Gustav Fischer, 1907).

60. Frosch, 58.

61. Otto Mugdan (Freisinnige Volkspartei), *SB* 165th Session (3.5.1911): 6329.

62. Wolff (1996), 91.

63. Reinhold Gerling in *NA* 26 (1898.): 188.

64. *NA* 1901 (11).

65. Apparently, Prießnitz packings were fairly common in treating vaccine-related outbreaks, abscesses, pustules, etc. HSta PK I. HA Rep. 76, *VIII B, 3926. "Aufklärungsblatt"* (1902).

66. *NA* 1901 (12).

67. Imperial Office of Health (1900), 92–93. The anti-vaccination associations did not just address the spectacular images to the public. One post card addressed to the Minister of the Interior in July 1909 showed 2 images side-by-side: one—the smaller image—a plump, blond boy. The larger one, a shriveled boy with two massive abscesses on his arms. The postcard was captioned: "One and 3/4 year old boy from Hanover, before vaccination, totally healthy, vaccinated 21 September, 1908, Hospital 7 October, 1908, died 18 October, 1908." It is unlikely that the post card had any effect on the ministry officials who received it (though it might have on the post handlers who delivered it, and it certainly did on this researcher). HSta PK I. HA Rep. 76, VIII B, 3926.

68. Kirchner *SB* 243rd Sitting (28.4.1914): 8310.

69. Whether or not Wegener was on target in his accounting, it is clear that he was a loose cannon, as indicated by the titles of some of his works. See, for example, *Impf-Friedhof. Was das Volk, die Sachverständigen und die Regierungen vom 'Segen der Impfung' wissen.* (Frankfurt am Main: Wegener, 1912); *Unerhört!!, Verteidigung und Angriff eines Staatsbürgers; Gegen Kirchner!* (Frankfurt am Main: Wegener, 1911).

70. Frosch, 58.

71. Kirchner (1911), 109, 11, 127. See also Kirchner, *SB* 243rd Session (28.4.1914): 8311. It was not only state-mandated defenders of the vaccine law that made these kinds of claims. Dr. Otto Mugdan (FsVP) made the same claim in his May 1911 address. Mugdan, *SB* 165th Session (3.5.1911): 6330. Wilhelm Arning (National Liberal) made similar comments in his 30 January 1911 address. Arning *SB* 117th Session (30.1.1911): 4278.

72. Report—President of the Imperial Office of Health to the Minister of the Interior, 25 June 1904. HSta PK IHA Rep. 76, VIII B, 3918.

73. Friedrich Blochmann, *Ist die Schutzpockenimpfung mit allen notwendigen Kautelen umgeben? Erörtert an einem mit Verlust des einen Auges verbundenen Falle von Vaccineübertragung* (Tübingen: F. Pietzker, 1904).

74. Report—President of the Imperial Office of Health to the Minister of the Interior, 25 June 1904. HSta PK IHA Rep. 76, VIII B, 3918.

75. Ibid.

76. The Blochmann case was reported not just in Germany, but in the United States as well. *St. Louis Medical Review*, March 17, 1906: 217–18.

77. A Berlin Police Inspector reported on one such case in January 1906. Charged with investigating Hugo Regel's failure to vaccinate his infant child, Police Inspector Cortemme reported that Regel's actions were not the result of bad intentions. It was, rather "the financial decline of the family" that was the reason for his oversight. As Cortemme reported it, it is difficult to imagine a more unfortunate story. In 1904, Hugo Regel suffered a broken leg which, because of improper treatment, failed to heal properly. The severe cramping that resulted from his accident made it impossible to continue as a laborer, and Regel had to give up his job in the milk trade. Now, he was selling artificial flowers on the streets. His wife made the flowers at home, but the income was barely three Marks per week. These were only some of their problems. On November 20, 1905, Regel's wife suffered a miscarriage and was still recovering her health. This was made difficult by their inability to purchase the nutrition-rich foods that would help her to regain her strength. Earning a living and feeding and housing two adults was already a challenge. But as Cortemme reported, the Regels had three children, all under the age of eight. Cortemme was investigating the family to determine whether or not they should be fined for their failure to vaccinate their youngest child. Given the circumstances, he recommended against it. I HA Rep. 76 Kultusministerium VIIIB Nr. 4011. Der Polizei-Präsident—Abteilung VI—Betrifft Gnadengesuch des Hugo Regel.

78. Paul Mirus, for example. For parliamentary comment, see Dr. Maximilian Pfeiffer (Center), *SB* 117th Session (30.2.1911): 4275.

79. Hermann Wolf, "Die Gesundheitspflege des Arbeiters, (II)," *NH* 13, no. 2

(1901): 12. Independent calculations by Voit and Lahmann put the figures much higher at Rm 766 and Rm 1095, respectively. For another contemporary account, see Dr. med. Georg Bonne, "Über die Notwendigkeit einer systematischen Dezentralisation unserer Großstädte in hygienischer, sozialer und volkswirtschaftlicher Beziehung." Part I, in *Monatsschrift für Soziale Medizin. Zentralblatt für die gesamte wissenschaftliche und praktische Sozialmedizin* 1, no. 8 (1904): 370.

80. Pfeiffer (Center), *SB* 117th Session (30.2.1911): 4275. Pfeiffer's remarks seem extraordinarily prescient. It was only decades later that public health officials working in the global south discovered that conditions on the ground differed dramatically from the antiseptic clinical environment where vaccinations would ideally be conducted.

81. Kirchner, *SB* 165th Session (3.5.1911): 6325. This figure is, surprisingly, a conservative estimate based on Ministry of Health data. Kirchner reported that roughly 3 million German children were vaccinated or revaccinated annually, and that between 12 and 13 % of eligible children were—legally or illegally—evading the vaccine mandate.

82. HSta PK I HA Rep. 76 Kultusministerium VIIIB Nr. 4009. District President to the Minister of the Interior (29.7.1891): "Die Beschwerde der Versicherungsbeamten Longino in Steglitz."

83. Ibid.

84. The case of retiree F. Butterbrodt from Hildesheim is another good example. Over a period of several years, Butterbrodt bombarded administrators of the vaccine regime with petitions to exempt his five children, ages 1–16, from compulsory vaccination. Administrators had little patience for these "fanatics," and Butterbrodt received no exception for his children. But even in such instances, bureaucrats and police officials were obliged to document the cases, correspond with petitioners and superiors, and enforce fines and potential jail terms. HSta PK I HA Rep. 76 Kultusministerium VIIIB Files 4008 and 4009 (1887–1896).

85. HSta PK I HA Rep. 76 Kultusministerium VIIIB Nr. 4010. Police report to the Minister of the Interior (18.3.1901).

86. Engl. translation: *Vaccination Law of April 8, 1874* (Berlin: B. Paul, 1904), 1. My emphasis.

87. Kirchner, 68. This meant that, in 1900, just 88.2 % of the population had been vaccinated or revaccinated.

88. HSta PK I HA Rep. 76 Kultusministerium VIIIB Nr. 4010. Police report to the Minister of the Interior (18.3.1901).

89. *NA* 26 (1898): 115.

90. *NA* 26 (1898): 188.

91. Engl. translation: *Vaccination Law of April 8, 1874* (Berlin: B. Paul, 1904). As per section 1 of the vaccine law, parents had to present their children for vaccination by Dec. 31 of the birth year. This meant that a child born on January 1 could defer vaccination for 364 days, a child born on July 1 could defer for 6 months, and so on. At the end of the year, parents could apply to a doctor for a deferral based on their child's health. Deferral, then, was as easy as being excused from school for the day—one

simply needed a doctor's note. The author of an educational pamphlet also told parents that "vaccine officials are neither obliged nor allowed to question the veracity of (such a document) from a licensed doctor." With almost no legal risk for parents or testifying doctors, the law made it possible to postpone vaccination for as much as two years. In some cases, it was possible to defer for much longer, especially if doctors would testify to chronic illness on the part of the vaccinee. HSta PK I. HA Rep. 76, Kultusministerium VIII B Nr. 3926. Aufklärungsblatt (1902).

92. HSta PK I. HA Rep. 76, Kultusministerium VIII B Nr. 3926. Aufklärungsblatt (1902).

93. Mirus, 5.

94. Pfeiffer, SB 165th Session (3.5.1911): 6316.

95. Deutsche Tageszeitung (18.09.1909) "Zum Impfgesetz."

96. Dr. Georg Burckhardt (Christian Social) SB 243rd Session (28.4.1914): 8289; Kirchner SB 243rd Session (28.4.1914): 8312.

97. Pfeiffer SB (3.5.1911): 6316.

98. "Zur Impffrage," Deutsche Tageszeitung: (14.12.1909). See also "Kann die Impfung der Kinder erzwungen werden?" NA 35 (1907): 38-9.

99. "Zur Impffrage," Deutsche Tageszeitung: (14.12.1909).

100. "Zur Kampf gegen den Impfzwang," NA 22 (1894): 7-10. The total numbers are as follows: 3 conservatives, 3 Reichspartei, 10 Antisemiten, 14 Zentrum, 3 National Liberale, 3 Freisinnige, 9 süddeutsche Volkstpartei, 39 Sozialdemokraten, 1 Elsasser, 1, Bauernbund.

101. In the 1898 legislative period, for example, there were only 5 doctors in the parliament out of a total of 397 representatives.

102. NA 26 (1898): 51.

103. NA 26 (1898): 221.

104. NA 26 (1898): 252.

105. Dr. Otto Fischbeck, SB 243rd Session (28.4.1914): 8303.

106. Michael Gross, The War Against Catholicism: Liberalism and the Anti-Catholic Imagination in Nineteenth-Century Germany (Ann Arbor: University of Michigan Press, 2004). On the politics of the Social Democratic Party, see Richard Breitman, "Negative Integration and Parliamentary Politics: Literature on German Social Democracy, 1890–1933," Central European History 13 (1980): 175–97.

107. HStaPK I. HA Rep. 76, Kultusministerium VIII B, 3926. Excerpt from the153rd Session (27.2.1902).

108. Pfeiffer, SB 117th Session (30.1.1911): 4274.

109. Ibid.

110. Ibid.

111. Ibid.

112. Ibid. Pfeiffer's Center Party colleague and cosponsor of the 1911 petition to review and revise the 1874 law, Martin Fassbender, made similar points. Fassbender, SB 165th Session (3.5.1911): 6329.

113. Volker Berghahn, for example, points out that although the state needed to secure parliamentary majorities to win approval of its budgets, Wilhelm II also had the power to dissolve parliament, to call new elections, and to proscribe parties. Even the

ability to control the budgets was partial. Parliament voted on military budgets only every five years. Volker Rolf Berghahn, *Germany and the Approach of War in 1914* (New York: St. Martin's Press, 1973), 10. In general, the historical consensus has pushed in a rather different direction, suggesting that perception of an impotent parliament was overblown. But as Josh Traficante has shown, parliamentary parties were forced to walk a fine line in their relationship with the state. Parliamentary opposition, in other words, was always fraught with danger: "In essence, while the Reichstag could and did modify government-sponsored bills, including military funding, the looming threat from the throne ensured that while concessions could be extracted, their extent was limited. The case of the Catholic Center Party as it operated in this system, in particular in its response to military spending bills, illustrates this dynamic." Joshua Traficante, "Walking the Line: The Center Party, the Reichstag, and Militarism in Imperial Germany, 1890–1906" (MA thesis: University of Chicago, 2010).

114. Pfeiffer, *SB* 117th Session (30.1.1911): 4276.

115. "Die Impffrage im preußischen Abgeordnetenhause." *NA* 41(1913): 124–27. Here, 125. In 1911, Kirchner described the activities of anti-vaccine activists as "almost criminal." Similarly, in dismissing criticisms from the well-known anti-vaccine activist Heinrich Molenaar in 1914, Kirchner claimed that he was mentally unstable. Kirchner, *SB* 243rd Session (28.4.1914): 8311.

116. HStaPK I. HA Rep. 76, VIII B, 3926. Excerpt from the parliamentary record. Friedrich Endemann (National Liberal) 153rd Session (27.2.1902).

117. Susan Pedersen, "Anti-Condescensionism. *Bodily Matters: The Anti-Vaccination Movement in England, 1853–1907*, by Nadja Durbach." Book review in *London Review of Books*, September 1, 2005: 1–9.

118. Ibid., 3.

119. Durbach, 201.

120. Maehle, 128.

121. Friedrich Thiele (Social Democrat) *SB* 165th Session (3.5.1911): 6311, 6313. This equation linking the medical establishment to the allegedly dogmatic authority of the church is already familiar from earlier chapters, and was frequently voiced by anti-vaccine activists. In 1883, for example, Dr. med. Eugen Bilfinger wrote, "It is only the doctors who swear by the vaccine dogma, who claim that it is not a matter for discussion." Eugen Bilfinger, *Ueber fuer und wider den Impfzwang* (Stuttgart: Kommissionsverlag von Konrad Wittwer, 1883), 9. Like Thiele, Bilfinger claimed that defenders of the 1874 law treated vaccination as though it was gospel, and not science. If this equation was common over a period of decades, something had changed in the years between Bilfinger's pamphlet and Thiele's speech. The critique of vaccination had moved from the medical margins to the center of the parliamentary floor.

122. Bock *SB* 243rd Session (28.4.1914): 8290.

123. HStaPK I. HA Rep. 76, VIII B, 3926. Excerpt from the parliamentary record. Max Liebermann von Sonnenberg (German Social Reform Party—Anti-Semite) *SB* 35th Session (17.2.1904). Interestingly, Liebermann von Sonnenberg was from Weißwasser in Saxony, where one of the "spectacular cases" mentioned earlier in this chapter took place.

124. Dr. Wilhelm Winsch, "Die Pocken im Deutschen Reich und in Oester-

reich-Ungarn während des Weltkrieges." *NA* 47 (1919): 121–22. Winsch claimed that poor hygiene and food scarcity were the key to understanding smallpox outbreaks during the war. After all, military men were, without exception, revaccinated upon entry into military service, and the civilian population was already, in large measure, vaccinated according to mandate established by the 1874 law. In the second part of this series, Winsch also notes that anti-vaccine agitation was banned in 1916 by the Military Governors General. Dr. Wilhelm Winsch, "Die Pocken im Deutschen Reich und in Oesterreich-Ungarn während des Weltkrieges. Part II." *NA* 47(9), 1919:139–41.

125. See, for example, Dr. von Nießen's three-part essay, "Wie schützt man sich vor den Bazillen?" *NA* 55 (1927): issues 6, 8, 9.

126. On dissatisfaction with bacteriology and on the growth of social hygiene after the '90s, see Paul Weindling, "From Germ Theory to Social Medicine: Public Health, 1880–1930, in Deborah Brunton, ed., *Medicine Transformed. Health, Disease and Society in Europe, 1800–1930* (Manchester: Manchester University Press, 2004).

127. *NA* 1912 (7), "Rationelles Vorgehen in der Impfzwangsfrage," 199–200.

CONCLUSION

1. The tendencies underway in chapters 3 and 4 persisted during the Weimar Republic, with the increasing institutionalization of *Naturheilkunde*'s theory and practice. Carsten Timmermann's work offers wonderful insights into this period. See his *Weimar Medical Culture: Doctors, Healers and the Crisis of Medicine in Interwar Germany, 1918–1933* (Diss: University of Manchester, 1999). For more on issues explored in chapter 2, see Florentine Fritzen.

2. Bundesleitung, *Fünfzig Jahre Arbeit für die Volksgesundheit. Festschrift zum fünfzigjährigen Bestehen des Deutschen Bundes für naturgemäße Lebens- und Heilweise* (Berlin, 1939). Gerhard Wagner.

3. Detlef Bothe, *Neue Deutsche Heilkunde* (Husum: Mathiessen, 1991); Alfred Haug, "'Neue Deutsche Heilkunde.' Naturheilkunde und 'Schulmedizin' im Nationalsozialismus," in Johanna Bleker and Norbert Jachertz, eds. *Medizin im Dritten Reich* (Cologne: Deutscher Ärzte Verlag, 1993); Uwe Heyll, *Wasser, Fasten, Luft und Licht. Die Geschichte der Naturheilkunde in Deutschland.* (Frankfurt: Campus Verlag, 2006); Robert Jütte, *Geschichte der alternativen Medizin : Von der Volksmedizin zu den unkonventionellen Therapien von Heute* (Munich: C. H. Beck, 1996).

4. Heyll, 232.

5. Ibid., 239.

6. Ibid., 265.

7. Ibid., 271. I have not confirmed this point independently, but the DDR did pursue a policy of eradicating so-called medical alternatives, including natural healing and homeopathy. Margaret Stacey, *Sociology of Health and Healing. A Textbook* (New York: Routledge, 1988), 155.

8. Ibid., 273.

9. Fritzen, passim.

BIBLIOGRAPHY

PRIMARY SOURCES

Archival Sources

Bundesarchiv—Berlin—Lichterfelde
Ministry of the Interior—(BA R/1501): 190130–190136. Files Pertaining to the Regulation of Quackery, 1899–1914.
Press Archives—(BA R/8034 II): 1807–1809. Files Pertaining to Medical Matters, 1908–1914.

Geheimes Staatsarchiv Preußischer Kulturbesitz—Berlin—Dahlem
Ministry of Health—(GstaPK I HA Rep 76 VIIIB): 1316–1317. Files Pertaining to Water, Diet, and Natural Therapies, 1874–1926.
Ministry of Health—(GstaPK I HA Rep 76 VIIIB): 1327–1333. Files Pertaining to the Practice of Healing by Laymen, 1894–1923.
Ministry of the Interior—(GstaPK IHA Rep 77 Tit 719): 26; (GstaPK IHA Rep 77 Tit 806): 5, 20, 37; (GstaPK IHA Rep 77 Tit 807): 5. Files Pertaining to the Oversight and Advancement of Natural Healing and Bathing Facilities, 1853–1921.

Humboldt Universitätsarchiv—Berlin
Medical Faculty—(HUA): 268, 296, 1386. Correspondence, 1919–1939.
Medical Faculty—(HUA): Universitäts Kurator Vols. 1–3. Files Pertaining to the Search for an Extraordinary Professor of Medicine, 1919–1920.

Sächsisches Hauptstaatsarchiv—Dresden
Ministry of the Interior—(HstaD): 15231. Files Pertaining to Quackery, 1884–1904.
Ministry of the Interior—(HstaD): 15232–15236. Files Pertaining to the Practice of Medicine by Nonlicensed Persons dated between 1904–1921.

Sächsisches Staatsarchiv—Leipzig
Police Presidium—(HstaL–PP-V): 74, 118, 310, 317, 492, 705, 1479, 1506, 1824, 2508, 2646, 2719, 4268. Files Pertaining to Registered Associations, 1901–1949.

Stadtarchiv Leipzig—Leipzig
Municipal Administration—(StdtL–Kap. 35): 383, 396, 417. 747, 779, 826, 915, 946, 990, 1145, 1297, 1807. Various Correspondence, 1884–1940.

Periodicals

Allgemeiner Beobachter. Halbmonatsschrift für alle Fragen des modernen Lebens.
Archiv für Physikalisch-diätetische Therapie in der ärztlichen Praxis. Offizielles Organ des Ärzte-Vereins für physikalisch-diätetische Therapie.
Archiv für soziale Medizin und Hygiene. (Neue Folge der Monatsschrift für Soziale Medizin.)
Blätter für Volksaufklärung: Monatsschrift der Gesellschaft für Volksaufklärung und ihrer Ortsgruppen.
Gesundheitslehrer. Volkstümliche Monatsschrift. Offizielles Organ der Deutschen Gesellschaft zur Bekämpfung des Kurpfuschertums.
Mehr Licht: Organ des Deutschen Bundes für Persönlichkeitskultur.
Der Naturarzt. Zeitschrift des Deutschen Bundes der Vereine für Gesundheitspflege und arzneilose Heilweise.
Die Neue Heilkunst. Volkstümliche Halbmonatsschrift für naturgemässe Gesundheitspflege, soziale Hygiene, Magnetismus, Hypnotismus und Seelenheilkunde.
Unsere Hausarzt. Wochenschrift für Gesundheitspflege, Naturheilkunde, und Lebenskunst.
Die Volksgesundheit. Zeitschriift des Verbandes der Vereine für Volksgesundheit.
Zeitschrift für diätetische und physikalische Therapie.

Published Works

Anon. *Der Kampf um die Augen-Diagnose. Stenographischer Bericht des Felke-Prozesses vor dem Landgericht Crefeld vom 27 Oktober bis 3. November 1909.* Crefeld: Verlag von Albert Fürst Nacht, 1909.
Anon. *Adolf Damaschke zu seinem 50. Geburtstage.* Franfurt Oder: TR Wotsch u. Sohn, 1915.
Anon. *Die Obstbausiedlung Eden in Oranienburg in den ersten 25 Jahren ihres Bestehens.* Oranienburg: Verlag der Obstabausiedlung Eden, 1920.
Baltzer, Eduard. *Ideen zur Socialen Reform. Sendschreiben an die Hochgeehrte Mexicanische Societät fur Geographie und Statistik in Mexico.* Nordhausen: Verlag Ferd. Fürstemann, 1873.
———. *Vegetarisches Kochbuch für Freunde der natürlichen Lebensweise.* Leipzig: Verlag von H. Hartung und Sohn, 1903.
———. *Erinnerungen. Bilder aus meinem Leben.* Frankfurt an Main: Verlag des deutschen Vegetarier-Bundes, 1907.
Bielau, Franz von. *Authentische Biographie von Schlesiens berühmten Naturarzt und Erfinder der Wasserheilkunde.* Freiwaldau: Verlag von Betty Titze, 1902.
Bilfinger, Eugen. *Wie ich Naturarzt Wurde.* Leipzig: Hartung Verlag, 1901.
Bilz, Friedrich Eduard. *Wie schafft man bessere Zeiten? Die wahre Lösung der sozi-*

alen Frage nach dem Naturgesetz. Dresden Radebeul: Verlag von F. E. Bilz, 1894.

———. *Das Neue Naturheilverfahren: Lehr und Nachschlagebuch der naturgemäßen Heilweise und Gesundheitspflege*. Leipzig: F. E. Bilz Verlag, 1898.

———. *Der Zukunftsstaat. Staatseinrichtung im Jahre 2000. Neue Weltanschauung. Jedermann wird ein glückliches und sorgenfreies Dasein gesichert*. Leipzig: F. E. Bilz Verlag, 1904.

Böing, Heinrich. *Tatsachen zur Pocken- und Impffrage. Eine statistisch-ätiologisch-kritische Studie*. Leipzig: Breitkopf & Härtel, 1882.

Bundesleitung. *25 Jahre im Dienste der Volksgesundheit. Festschrift zum 25 jährigen Bestehen des Deutschen Bundes der Vereine für naturgemässe Lebens- und Heilweise*. Berlin: Eigener Verlag, 1914.

Bundesleitung. *Fünfzig Jahre Arbeit für die Volksgesundheit. Festschrift zum fünfzigjährigen Bestehen des Deutschen Bundes für naturgemäße Lebens- und Heilweise*. Berlin: Eigener Verlag, 1939.

Damschke, Adolf. *Manchestertum, Anti-Semitismus, oder Bodenbesitzreform*. Berlin: Thormann & Goetsch, 1891.

———. *Die Organisation der deutschen Naturheilbewegung*. Berlin: Verlag von Wilhelm Möller, 1896.

———. *Was ist National-Sozial?* Berlin: Verlag der 'Hilfe,' 1898.

———. *Die Bodenreform: Grundsätzliches und Geschichtliches zur Erkenntnis und Überwinding der sozialen Not*. 15th ed. Jena: Verlag von Gustav Fischer, 1918.

Gerling, Walter. *Reinhold Gerling. Sein Leben und Wirken. Biographische Skizze mit 3 Abbildungen*. Oranienburg: Orania Verlag, 1923.

Gleich, Lorenz. *Nur Kein Wasser! Beiträge zur Begründung der Wasserheillehre in einer Sammlung von Aufsätzen von Dr. Gleich, Wasserarzt in München*. Edited by B. Vanoni. Augsburg: Verlag von Lampart & Comp, 1847.

———. *Ueber die Nothwendigkeit einer Reform der sogenannten Hydrotherapie, oder Geist und Bedeutung der Schrothlichen Heilweise. Nebst einem kurzen Reisebericht als Einleitung*. Munich: Johann Deschler, 1851.

Hahn, Theodor. *Die Ritter vom Fleische. Offene Briefe über die Ernährungsfrage an Prof. Dr. med. Virchow, Voit, Liebig, Bock Moleschott et al*. Berlin: Theobald Grieben, 1869.

———. *Der Vegetarismus, seine wissenschaftliche Begründung und seine Bedeutung für das leibliche, geistige und sittliche Wohl des Einzelnen, wie der gesammten Menschheit. Ein Beitrag zur Lösung der sozialen Frage*. Berlin: Theobald Grieben, 1869.

———. *Praktisches Handbuch der naturgemäßen Heilweise*, Vol. 1. Berlin: Theobald Grieben, 1870.

Hammer, Walter. *Lebensreform und Politik*. Berlin: Verlag Lebensreform, 1910.

Held-Ritt, Ernst von. *Prißnitz auf Gräfenberg oder treue Darstellung seines Heilverfahrens mit kaltem Wasser*. 1837. Reprint, Würzburg: Bergstadtverlag Wilhelm Gottlieb Korn, 1988.

Hennemann, H. *Das Sündenregister der Medicinheilkunde*. 2nd ed. St. Gallen: Verlag von Altweg-Weber zu Kreuzberg, 1875.

———. *Die Impfvergiftung der Jugend des deutschen Reichs.* 1875—no publication data.

Horsfall, T. C. *The Improvement of the Dwellings and Surroundings of the People. The Example of Germany.* Manchester: University Press, 1904.

Imperial Office of Health. *Blattern und Schutzpockenimpfung. Denkschrift zur Beurtheilung des Nutzens des Impfgesetzes vom 8. April 1874 und zur Würdigung der dagegen gerichteten Angriffe.* Berlin: Julius Springer, 1900.

Just, Adolf. *Kehrt zur Natur Züruck! Die Wahre naturgemäße Heil—und Lebensweise, Wasser, Licht, Luft, Erde, Früchte und Wirkliches Christentum.* 1895. Rev. ed. Jungborn: Jungborn Verlag, 1910.

Kirchner, Martin. *Schutzpockenimpfung und Impfgesetz.* Berlin: Richard Schoeß, 1911.

Kraepelin, Emil. *100 Years of Psychiatry.* Translated by Wade Baskins. New York: Philosophical Library, Inc., 1962.

Mirus, Paul. *Die Impffrage und der Verband deutscher Impfgegner.* Dortmund: Verlag von Robert Keßler, 1910.

Molenaar, Heinrich. *Impfschutz und Impfgefahren.* Munich: Melchior Kupferschmid, 1912.

Munde, Carl. *Memoiren eines Wasserarztes,* Vol. 1. 2nd ed. Dresden & Leipzig: in der Arnoldischen Buchhandlung, 1847.

Nittinger, C. G. G. *Die Impfung ein Mißbrauch.* Stuttgart: Emil Ebner, 1867.

Rausse, J. H. *Anleitung zur Ausübung der Wasser -oder Naturheilkunde für Jedermann, der zu Lesen Versteht.* 4th ed. Leipzig: Gesundheitsblätter Verlag, 1895.

Rikli, Arnold. *Die Grundlehre der Naturheilkunde einschließlich die atmosphärische Cur. 'Es Werde Licht.'* Leipzig: L. Fernau Verlag, 1895.

Schlegel, Emil. *Die Augendiagnose des Dr. Ignaz von Peczély.* Tübingen: Verlag von Franz Fues, 1906.

Schönenberger, Franz. *Lebenskunst—Heilkunst. Ärztlicher Ratgeber für Gesunde und Kranke.* Zwickau: Förster & Borries Verlag, 1906.

Seefeld, Alfred von. *Studien über Gesundheit und Krankheit.* Berlin: Theobald Grieben, 1869.

Simons, Gustav. *Die Überwindung des Kapitalismus. Eine Vorbedingung für die Volksgesundheit.* Oranienburg bei Berlin: Verlag des Deutschen Kulturbundes für Politik, 1913.

———.*Das Gesamtbild deutscher Erneuerungsbestrebungen. Ein Leitfaden für alle Reformer, besonders für die Führer.* Oranienburg: Wilhelm Möller, 1913.

Walde, Philo vom. *Vincenz Prießnitz: Sein Leben und Sein Wirken. Zur Gedenkfeier seines Hundertsten Geburtstages dargestellt.* Berlin: Verlag von Wilhelm Möller, 1899.

Weber, Adolf. *Die Großstadt und ihre sozialen Probleme.* Leipzig: Quelle & Meyer, 1908.

Wehberg, Heinrich. *Die Bodenreform im Lichte des Humanistischen Sozialismus.* München und Leipzig: Duncker & Humblot, 1913.

Winsch, Wilhelm. *Wie ich Naturarzt wurde! ein ärztliches Glaubensbekenntnis nach einem im Bürgersaal des Berliner Rathauses gehaltenen Vortrag: mit einem Nachwort über die drohende Aufhebung der Kurierfreiheit.* Berlin: Lebenskunst-Heilkunst, 1910.

Wrede, Richard, and Reinfels, Hans von. *Das Geistige Berlin: eine Enzyklopädie des geistigen Lebens Berlins.* Vol. 1. Berlin: Verlag von Hugo Storm, 1897.

SECONDARY SOURCES

Allen, Arthur. *Vaccine. The Controversial Story of Medicine's Greatest Lifesaver.* New York: W. W. Norton & Co., 2007.

Barlösius, Eva. *Naturgemässe Lebensführung: zur Geschichte der Lebensreform um die Jahrhundertwende.* Frankfurt: Campus Verlag, 1997.

Baumgardt, M., and R. Dose, eds. *Magnus Hirschfeld—Leben und Werk Ausstellungskatalog aus Anlaß seines 50. Todestags.* Hamburg: Bockel Verlag, 1992.

Baumgarten, Judith. "Erbau dein Heim auf freiem Grund! Bodenreform und Siedlungsidee: Adolf Damaschke und die Siedlungsgenossenschaft Eden-Oranienburg." In *Adolf Damaschke und Henry George: Ansätze zu einer Theorie und Politik der Bodenreform,* edited by Klaus Hugler and Hans Diefenbacher. Marburg: Metropolis Verlag, 2005.

Baxby, Derrick. *Small Pox Vaccine, Ahead of Its Time. How the Late Development of Laboratory Methods and Other Vaccines Affected the Acceptance of Smallpox Vaccine.* Berkeley: The Jenner Museum, 2001.

Bazin, Hervé. *The Eradication of Smallpox. Edward Jenner and the First and Only Eradication of a Human Infectious Disease.* Translated by Andrew Morgan and Glenise Morgan. New York: Academic Press, 2000.

Bergmann, Klaus. *Agrarromantik und Großstadtfeindschaft.* Meisenheim am Glan: Hain, 1970.

Bhattacharya, S., M. Harrison, and M. Worboys, eds. *Fractured States: Smallpox, Public Health and Vaccination Policy in British India, 1800–1947.* Hyderabad: Orient Longman Private Limited, 2005.

Blackbourn, David, and Geoff Eley. *The Peculiarities of German History: Bourgeois Society and Politics in Nineteenth-Century Germany.* New York: Oxford University Press, 1984.

Bothe, Detlef. *Neue Deutsche Heilkunde.* Husum: Mathiessen, 1991.

Brauchle, Alfred. *Die Geschichte der Naturheilkunde in Lebensbildern.* Stuttgart: Reclam Verlag, 1951.

———. *Zur Geschichte der Physiotherapie. Naturheilkunde in ärztlichen Lebensbildern.* Heidelberg: Haug Verlag, 1971.

Brederlow, Jorn. *'Lichtfreunde' und 'Freie Gemeinden.' Religiöser Protest und Freiheitsbewegungen im Vormärz und in der Revolution von 1848/49.* Munich: Oldenbourg Verlag, 1976.

Broman, Thomas. *The Transformation of German Academic Medicine, 1750–1820.* Cambridge: Cambridge University Press, 1996.

Browne, Janet. "Spas and Sensibilities: Darwin at Malvern." In *The Medical History of Waters and Spas,* ed. Roy Porter, 102–13. London: Wellcome Institute for the History of Medicine, 1990.

Brunton, Deborah. "Dealing with Disease in Populations: Public Health, 1830–1880." In *Medicine Transformed: Health, Disease and Society in Europe, 1800–1930*, ed. Deborah Brunton. Manchester: Manchester University Press, 2004.

Buchholz, Kai, et al., eds. *Die Lebensreform: Entwürfe zur Neugestaltung von Leben und Kunst um 1900*. Two volumes: Darmstadt: Institut Mathildenhöhe–Häusser, 2001.

Bullock, N., and J. Read. *The Movement for Housing Reform in Germany and France, 1840–1914*. Cambridge: Cambridge University Press, 1985.

Bynum, W. F., and Roy Porter, eds. *Medical Fringe and Medical Orthodoxy, 1750–1850*. London: Croom Helm, 1987.

Cocks, Geoffrey, and Konrad Jarausch, eds. *German Professions, 1800–1950*. New York: Oxford University Press, 1990.

Conti, Christoph. *Abschied vom Bürgertum: Alternative Bewegungen in Deutschland von 1890 bis heute*. Reinbek bei Hamburg: Rowohlt Verlag, 1984.

Cooter, Roger, and Stephen Pumfrey. "Separate Spheres and Public Places: Reflections on the History of Science Popularization and Science in Popular Culture." Cited in *History of Science* 22 (1994): 237–67.

Crosland, Maurice. "The *Officiers de Santé* of the French Revolution: A Case Study in the Changing Language of Medicine." *Medical History* 48 (2004): 229–44.

Daum, Andreas. *Wissenschaftspopularisierung im 19. Jahrhundert: Bürgerliche Kultur, Naturwissenschaftliche Bildung und die deutsche Öffentlichkeit, 1848–1914*. Munich: R. Oldenbourg Verlag, 1998.

Dear, Peter. *The Intelligibility of Nature: How Science Makes Sense of the World*. Chicago: University of Chicago Press, 2006.

Dietrich, Isolde. *Hammer, Zirkel, Gartenzaum. Die Politik der SED gegenüber den Kleingärtnern*. Berlin: BoD, 2003.

Donegan, Jane. "*Hydropathic Highway to Health.*" *Women and Water-Cure in Antebellum America*. Westport: Greenwood Press, 1986.

Durbach, Nadja. *Bodily Matters. The Anti-Vaccination Movement in England, 1853–1907*. Durham: Duke University Press, 2005.

Eley, Geoff, and James Retallack, eds. *Wilhelminism and Its Legacies: German Modernities, Imperialism, and the Meanings of Reform, 1890–1930*. New York: Berghahn Books, 2003.

Engelhardt, Dietrich von. "Kausalität und Konditionalität in der modernen Medizin." In *Pathogenese: Grundzüge und Perspektiven einer Theoretischen Pathologie*, ed. Heinrich Schipperges, 32–58. Berlin: Springer Verlag, 1985.

Fraunholz, Uwe. *Motorphobia: Anti-automobiler Protest in Kaiserreich und Weimarer Republik*. Göttingen: Vandenhoeck & Ruprecht, 2002.

Fritzen, Florentine. *Gesünder Leben: Die Lebensreformbewegung im 20. Jahrhundert*. Stuttgart: Franz Steiner Verlag, 2006.

Galison, Peter, and Bruce Hevly. *Big Science: The Growth of Large-Scale Research*. Stanford: Stanford University Press, 1992.

Gevitz, Norman, ed. *Other Healers: Unorthodox Medicine in America*. Baltimore: Johns Hopkins University Press, 1988.

Geyer, M., and K. Jarausch. *Shattered Past: Reconstructing German Histories.* Princeton: Princeton University Press, 2003.

Gieryn, Thomas. *Cultural Boundaries of Science: Credibility on the Line.* Chicago: University of Chicago Press, 1999.

Gilman, Sander. *Franz Kafka.* London: Reaktion, 2005.

Goldberg, Ann. *Sex, Religion, and the Making of Modern Madness: The Eberbach Asylum and German Society, 1815–1849.* New York: Oxford University Press, 1999.

Goldstein, Jan. *The Post-Revolutionary Self: Politics and Psyche in France.* Cambridge, MA: Harvard University Press, 2005.

Green, Martin. *Mountain of Truth. The Counterculture Begins, 1900–1920.* Hanover: University of New England Press, 1986.

Gross, Michael. *The War Against Catholicism. Liberalism and the Anti-Catholic Imagination in Nineteenth-Century Germany.* Ann Arbor: University of Michigan Press, 2004.

Harlander, Tilman. "Zentralität und Dezentralisierung—Großstadtentwicklung und städtbauliche Leitbilder im 20. Jahrhundert." In *Zentralität und Raumgefüge der Großstädte im 20. Jahrhundert,* ed. Clemens Zimmermann, 23–40. Stuttgart: Franz Steiner Verlag, 2006.

Hau, Michael. *The Cult of Health and Beauty in Germany: A Social History, 1890–1930.* Chicago: University of Chicago Press, 2003.

Haug, Alfred. "'Neue Deutsche Heilkunde.' Naturheilkunde und 'Schulmedizin' im Nationalsozialismus." In *Medizin im Dritten Reich,* edited by Johanna Bleker and Norbert Jachertz. Cologne: Deutscher Ärzte Verlag, 1993.

Helfricht, Jürgen. *Friedrich Eduard Bilz. 1842–1922. Altmeister der Naturheilkunde in Sachsen.* Radebeul: Sinalco AG Detmold und Stadtverwaltung Radebeul, 1992.

———. *Vincenz Prießnitz (1799–1851) und die Rezeption seiner Hydrotherapie bis 1918. Ein Beitrag zur Geschichte der Naturheilbewegung.* Husum: Matthiesen, 2006.

Helmstädter, Axel, "Zur Geschichte der deutschen Impfgegnerbewegung," *Geschichte der Pharmazie* 42 (1990): 19–23.

Hentschel, R. F. *Franz Schönenberger, 1865–1933. Biobibliographie eines ärztlichen Vertreters der Naturheilkunde.* Med. Diss., Ludwig-Maximilians Universität, 1979.

Hessenbruch, Arne. "Science as Public Sphere: X-Rays Between Spiritualism and Physics." In *Wissenschaft und Öffentlichkeit in Berlin, 1870–1930,* ed. Constantin Goschlar. Stuttgart: Franz Steiner Verlag, 2000.

Heyll, Uwe. *Wasser, Fasten, Luft und Licht. Die Geschichte der Naturheilkunde in Deutschland.* Frankfurt: Campus Verlag, 2006.

Hubenstorf, M. "Alfred Grotjahn." In *Berlinische Lebensbilder: Mediziner,* ed. W. Treue and R. Winau, 337–58. Berlin: Colloquium Verlag, 1987.

Hübinger, Gangolf, ed. *Versammlungsort moderner Geister. Der Eugen-Diederichs-Verlag—Aufbruch ins Jahrhundert der Extreme.* Munich: Diederichs, 1996.

Huerkamp, Claudia. *Der Aufstieg der Ärzte im 19. Jahrhundert. Vom gelehrten Stand* zum Professionellen Experten. Das Beispiel Preußens. Göttingen: Vandenhoeck und Ruprecht. 1985.

———. "Medizinische Lebensreform im späten 19. Jahrhundert: Die Naturheilbewegung als Protest gegen die naturwissenschaftliche Universitätsmedizin." Vierteljahresschrift für Sozial und Wirtschaftsgeschichte 73 (1986): 158–82.

Institute of Medicine of the National Academies. The Smallpox Vaccination Program. Public Health in an Age of Terrorism [sic]. Washington: National Academies Press, 2001.

Jütte, Robert. Geschichte der alternativen Medizin: Von der Volksmedizin zu den unkonventionellen Therapien von Heute. Munich: C. H. Beck, 1996.

Jütte, Robert, ed. Geschichte der deutschen Ärzteschaft. Köln: Deutscher Ärzte-Verlag, 1997.

Katsch, Günter. Deutsches Museum der Kleingartenbewegung Leipzig: Kleingärten und Kleingärtner im 19. und 20. Jahrhundert. Leipzig: Sächsische Landesstelle für Museumswesen, 1996.

King, Lester. The Medical World of the Eighteenth Century. Chicago: University of Chicago Press, 1958.

Knorr-Cetina, Karin. Epistemic Cultures: How the Sciences Make Knowledge. Cambridge, MA: Harvard University Press, 1999.

Krabbe, Wolfgang. Gesellschaftsveränderung durch Lebensreform: Strukturmerkmale einer sozialreformerischen Bewegung im Deutschland der Industrialisierungsperiode. Göttingen: Vandenhoeck & Ruprecht, 1974.

Krizek, Vladimir. Kulturgeschichte des Heilbades. Leipzig: W. Kohlhammer, 1990.

Labisch, Alfons, "Doctors, Workers, and the Scientific Cosmology of the Industrial World: The Social Construction of 'Health' and 'Homo Hygienicus.'" Journal of Contemporary History 20 (1985): 599–615.

Ladd, Brian. Urban Planning and Civic Order in Germany, 1860–1914. Cambridge, MA: Harvard University Press, 1990.

Latour, Bruno. The Pasteurization of France. Translated by Alan Sheridan and John Law. Cambridge, MA: Harvard University Press, 1988.

———. Pandora's Hope: Essays on the Reality of Science Studies. Cambridge, MA: Harvard University Press, 1999.

Latour, Bruno, and Steve Woolgar. Laboratory Life: The Social Construction of Scientific Facts. Beverly Hills: Sage, 1979.

Lees, Andrew. Cities, Sin, and Social Reform in Imperial Germany. Ann Arbor: University of Michigan Press, 2002.

Lekan, Thomas, and Thomas Zeller, eds. Germany's Nature: Cultural Landscapes and Environmental History. New Brunswick, NJ: Rutgers University Press, 2005.

Lempa, Heikki. "The Spa: Emotional Economy and Social Classes in Nineteenth-Century Pyrmont." Central European History 35 (2002): 37–73.

———. Beyond the Gymnasium. Educating the Middle-Class Bodies in Classical Germany. New York: Lexington Books, 2007.

Lindemann. Mary. Health and Healing in Eighteenth Century Germany. Baltimore: Johns Hopkins University Press, 1996.

Linse, Ulrich. *Barfüssige Propheten. Erlöser der zwanziger Jahre*. Berlin: Siedler Verlag, 1983.

———. *Ökopax und Anarchie: eine Geschichte der ökologischen Bewegungen in Deutschland*. München: Deutscher Taschenbuch Verlag, 1986.

Lupton, Deborah. *Medicine as Culture. Illness, Disease, and the Body in Western Societies*. London: Sage Books, 2003.

Mackaman, Douglas. *Leisure Settings: Bourgeois Culture, Medicine, and the Spa in Modern France*. Chicago: University of Chicago Press, 1998.

Maehle, Andreas Holger. "Präventivmedizin als wissenschaftliches und gesellschaftliches Problem: Der Streit uber das Reichsimpfgesetz von 1874." *Medizin, Gesellschaft und Geschichte* 9 (1990): 127–48.

Matthäi, Ingrid. "Kleingartenbewegung und Arbeitergesundheit." *Medizin, Gesellschaft und Geschichte* 13 (1994): 189–206.

Melzer, Jörg. *Vollwerternährung: Diätetik, Naturheilkunde, Nationalsozialismus, sozialer Anspruch*. Stuttgart: Franz Steiner Verlag, 2003.

Mergel, Thomas. *Parlamentarische Kultur in der Weimarer Republik. Politische Kommunikation, symbolische Politik und Öffentlichkeit im Reichstag*. Düsseldorf: Droste, 2002.

Mosse, George. *The Crisis of German Ideology: Intellectual Origins of the Third Reich*. New York: Schocken Books, 1981.

Obst, Helmut. *Karl August Lingner. Ein Volkswohltäter? Kulturhistorische Studie anhand der Lingner-Bombastus Prozesse, 1906–1911*. Göttingen: V & R Unipress, 2005.

Ohl, A. H. T. H. *Der Einfluß Jean-Jacques Rousseaus (1712–1778) auf die deutsche Naturheilbewegung des 19. Jahrhunderts*. Med. Diss.: Ruhr Universität Bochum, 2005.

Oreskes, Naomi, and Erik Conway. *Merchants of Doubt: How a Handful of Scientists Obscured the Truth on Issues from Tobacco Smoke to Global Warming*. New York: Bloomsbury, 2010.

Payer, Lynn. *Medicine and Culture. Varieties of Treatment in the United States, England, West Germany, and France*. New York: Henry Holt, 1988.

Pickstone, John. *Ways of Knowing. A New History of Science, Technology and Medicine*. Chicago: University of Chicago Press, 2001.

Polanyi, Karl. *The Great Transformation. The Political and Economic Origins of Our Times*. Boston: Beacon Press, 2001.

Porter, Roy, ed. *The Medical History of Waters and Spas*. London: Wellcome Institute for the History of Medicine, 1990.

Porter, Theodore. *Trust in Numbers. The Pursuit of Objectivity in Science and Public Life*. Princeton: Princeton University Press, 1995.

Rabson, S. Milton. "Alfred Grotjahn, Founder of Social Hygiene." *Bulletin of the New York Academy of Medicine* 12 (1936): 43–58.

Ramsey, Matthew. *Professional and Popular Medicine in France, 1770–1830: The Social World of Medical Practice*. Cambridge: Cambridge University Press, 1998.

Regin, Cornelia. "Naturheilkunde und Naturheilbewegung im Deutschen Kaiserreich. Geschichte, Entwicklung und Probleme eines Bündnisses zwischen professionellen Laienpraktikern und Laienbewegung." *Medizin, Gesellschaft und Geschichte* 11 (1992): 177–202.

———. *Selbsthilfe und Gesundheitspolitik. Die Naturheilbewegung im Kaiserreich, 1889–1914*. Stuttgart: Franz Steiner Verlag, 1995.

Repp, Kevin. *Reformers, Critics, and the Paths of German Modernity: Anti-politics and the Search for Alternatives, 1890–1914*. Cambridge, MA: Harvard University Press, 2000.

Richards, Robert. *The Romantic Conception of Life: Science and Philosophy in the Age of Goethe*. Chicago: University of Chicago Press, 2002.

Ries, Elisabeth. "Monte Verità, Ascona: Oberfläche und Unterströmungen am Berg der Wahrheit." In *Pioniere, Poeten, Professoren. Eranos und der Monte Verità in der Zivilisationsgeschichte des 20. Jahrhunderts*, ed. Elisabetta Borone, Matthias Riedl, und Alexandra Tischel, 21–32. Würzburg: Königshausen & Neumann, 2004.

Rodenstein, Marianne. *Mehr Licht, mehr Luft: Gesundheitskonzepte im Städtebau seit 1750*. Frankfurt am Main: Campus Verlag, 1988.

Rohkrämer, Thomas. *Eine andere Moderne: Zivilisationskritik, Natur und Technik in Deutschland, 1880–1930*. Paderborn: Schöningh Verlag, 1999.

Rothschuh, Karl Eduard. "Die Konzeptualisierung der Naturheilkunde im 19. Jahrhundert." *Gesnerus* (1/2) 1981: 175–90.

———. *Naturheilbewegung, Reformbewegung, Alternativbewegung*. Stuttgart: Hippokrates Verlag, 1983.

Saler, Michael. "Modernity and Enchantment: A Historiographic Review." *American Historical Review* 111 (2006): 692–716.

Sarasin, Philipp. *Reizbare Maschinen. Eine Geschichte des Körpers, 1765–1914*. Frankfurt am Main: Suhrkamp, 2001.

Schlich, Thomas, and Ulrich Tröhler, eds. *The Risks of Medical Innovation. Risk Perception and Assessment in Historical Context*. London: Routledge, 2006.

Scholz, Joachim Joe. *"Haben wir die Jugend, so haben wir die Zukunft." Die Obstbausiedlung Eden/Oranienburg als alternatives Gesellschafts- und Erziehungsmodell (1896–1936)*. Berlin: Weidler Buchverlag, 2002.

Scull, Andrew. *Museums of Madness: The Social Organization of Insanity in Nineteenth Century England*. New York: St. Martin's, 1979.

Shapin, Steve. *A Social History of Truth: Civility and Science in Seventeenth Century England*. Chicago: University of Chicago Press, 1994.

———. "Science and the Public." In *Companion to the History of Modern Science*, ed. R. C. Olby, G. N. Castor, et al., 900–1006. London: Routledge, 1996.

Spitzer, Giselher. *Der Deutschen Naturismus, Idee und Entwicklung einer volkserzieherischen Bewegung im Schnittfeld von Lebensreform, Sport und Politik*. Ahrensburg bei Hamburg: I. Czwalina, 1983.

Spree, Reinhard. *Soziale Ungleichheit vor Krankheit und Tod: zur Sozialgeschichte des Gesundheitsbereichs im Deutschen Kaiserreich*. Göttingen: Vandenhoeck & Ruprecht, 1981.

———. "Kurpfuscherei-Bekämpfung und ihre sozialen Funktionen." In *Medizinische Deutungsmacht in sozialen Wandel des 19 und frühen 20. Jahrhunderts,* edited by Alfons Labisch and Reinhard Spree, 103–123. Bonn: Psychiatrie-Verlag, 1989.

Stern, Bernhard. *Should We Be Vaccinated? A Survey of the Controversy in Its Historical and Scientific Aspects.* New York: Harper & Brothers, 1927.

Stern, Fritz. *The Politics of Cultural Despair: A Study in the Rise of the Germanic Ideology.* Berkeley: University of California Press, 1961.

Sweeney, Dennis. "Reconsidering the Modernity Paradigm: Reform Movements, the Social and the State in Wilhelmine Germany." *Social History* 31 (2006): 405–34.

Terlinden, Ulla, and Susanna von Oertzen. *Die Wohnungsfrage ist Frauensache! Frauenbewegung und Wohnreform 1870–1933.* Berlin: Dietrich Reimer, 2006.

Teuteberg, Hans-Jürgen. "Zur Sozialgeschichte des Vegetarismus." *Vierteljahrschrift für Sozial und Wirtschaftsgeschichte* 81 (1994): 33–65.

Timmermann, Carsten. *Weimar Medical Culture: Doctors, Healers and the Crisis of Medicine in Interwar Germany, 1918–1933.* PhD diss: University of Manchester, 1999.

———. "Rationalizing 'Folk Medicine' in Interwar Germany: Faith, Business, and Science at 'Dr. Madaus & Co.'" *Social History of Medicine* 14 (2001): 459–82.

Treitel, Corinna. *A Science for the Soul: Occultism and the Genesis of the German Modern.* Baltimore: Johns Hopkins University Press, 2004.

———. "Max Rubner and the Biopolitics of Rational Nutrition." *Central European History* 41 (2008): 1–25.

Vigarello, Georges. *Concepts of Cleanliness: Changing Attitudes in France Since the Middle Ages.* Translated by Jean Birrell. Cambridge: Cambridge University Press, 1988.

Weindling, Paul. *Health, Race and German Politics Between National Unification and Nazism, 1870–1945.* Cambridge: Cambridge University Press, 1989.

Whorton, James. *Nature Cures. The History of Alternative Medicine in America.* Oxford: Oxford University Press, 2002.

Williams, John. *Turning to Nature in Germany: Hiking, Nudism, and Conservation, 1900–1940.* Stanford: Stanford University Press, 2007.

Williams, Raymond. "Ideas of Nature." In *Nature: Critical Concepts in the Social Sciences,* ed. John Bone, David Inglis, and Rhoda Wilkie, 47–63. New York: Routledge, 2005.

Witzler, Beate. *Großstadt und Hygiene: Kommunale Gesundheitspolitik in der Epoche der Urbanisierung.* Stuttgart: Franz Steiner Verlag, 1995.

Wolff, Eberhard. "Kultivierte Natürlichkeit: zum Naturbegriff der Naturheilbewegung." *Jahrbuch des Instituts für Geschichte der Medizin der Robert Bosch Stiftung* 6 (1986): 219–36.

———. "Medizinkritik der Impfgegner im Spannungsfeld zwischen Lebenswelt und Wissenschaftsorientierung." In *Medizinkritische Bewegungen im Deutschen Reich* (*ca. 1870–ca. 1933*), ed. Martin Dinges, 79–108. Stuttgart: Franz Steiner Verlag, 1996.

———. *Einschneidende Massnahmen. Pockenschutzimpfung und traditionale Gesellschaft im Württemberg des frühen 19. Jahrhunderts.* Stuttgart: Franz Steiner Verlag, 1998.

Zimmermann, Andrew. "Science and *Schaulust* in the Berlin Museum for Ethnology." In *Wissenschaft und Öffentlichkeit in Berlin, 1870–1930*, ed. Constantin Goschlar, 65–88. Stuttgart: Franz Steiner Verlag, 2000.

Zimmermann, Clemens. *Von der Wohnfrage zur Wohnungspolitik: Die Reformbewegung in Deutschland, 1845–1914.* Göttingen: Vandenhoeck & Ruprecht, 1991.

INDEX